FREE Study Skills Videos Offer

Dear Customer,

Thank you for your purchase from Mometrix! We consider it an honor and a privilege that you have purchased our product and we want to ensure your satisfaction.

As a way of showing our appreciation and to help us better serve you, we have developed Study Skills Videos that we would like to give you for FREE. These videos cover our *best practices* for getting ready for your exam, from how to use our study materials to how to best prepare for the day of the test.

All that we ask is that you email us with feedback that would describe your experience so far with our product. Good, bad, or indifferent, we want to know what you think!

To get your FREE Study Skills Videos, email freevideos@mometrix.com with *FREE STUDY SKILLS Videos* in the subject line and the following information in the body of the email:

- The name of the product you purchased.
- Your product rating on a scale of 1-5, with 5 being the highest rating.
- Your feedback. It can be long, short, or anything in between. We just want to know your impressions and experience so far with our product. (Good feedback might include how our study material met your needs and ways we might be able to make it even better. You could highlight features that you found helpful or features that you think we should add.)

If you have any questions or concerns, please don't hesitate to contact me directly.

Thanks again!

Sincerely,

Jay Willis
Vice President
jay.willis@mometrix.com
1-800-673-8175

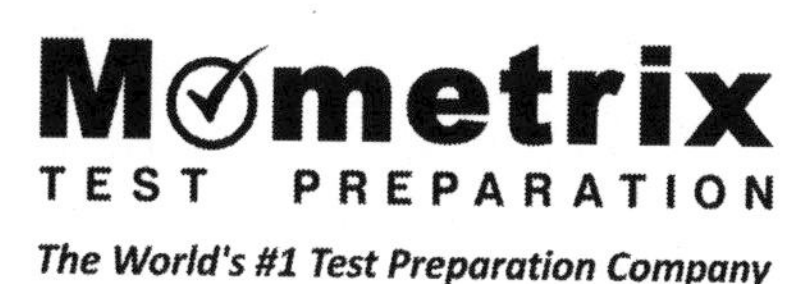

Secrets of the

PTCB Exam SECRETS

Study Guide

Your Key to Exam Success

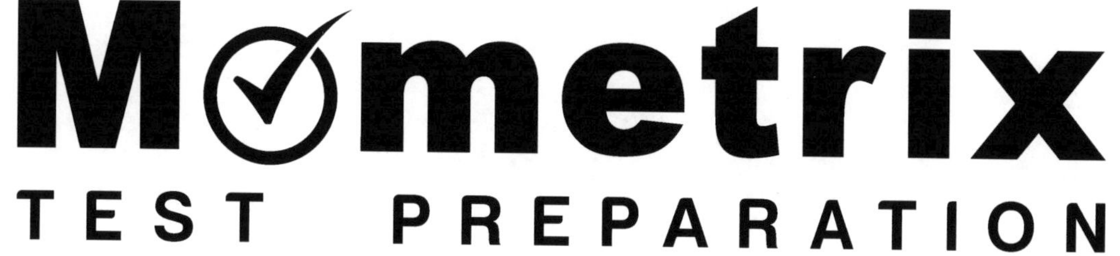

Written and edited by the Mometrix Pharmacy Tech Certification Test Team

Printed in the United States of America

This paper meets the requirements of ANSI/NISO Z39.48-1992 (Permanence of Paper).

Paperback
ISBN 13: 978-1-61072-799-0
ISBN 10: 1-61072-799-1

Ebook
ISBN 13: 978-1-62120-323-0
ISBN 10: 1-62120-323-9

Hardback
ISBN 13: 978-1-5167-0538-2
ISBN 10: 1-5167-0538-6

Dear Future Exam Success Story

First of all, **THANK YOU** for purchasing Mometrix study materials!

Second, congratulations! You are one of the few determined test-takers who are committed to doing whatever it takes to excel on your exam. **You have come to the right place.** We developed these study materials with one goal in mind: to deliver you the information you need in a format that's concise and easy to use.

In addition to optimizing your guide for the content of the test, we've outlined our recommended steps for breaking down the preparation process into small, attainable goals so you can make sure you stay on track.

We've also analyzed the entire test-taking process, identifying the most common pitfalls and showing how you can overcome them and be ready for any curveball the test throws you.

Standardized testing is one of the biggest obstacles on your road to success, which only increases the importance of doing well in the high-pressure, high-stakes environment of test day. Your results on this test could have a significant impact on your future, and this guide provides the information and practical advice to help you achieve your full potential on test day.

Your success is our success

We would love to hear from you! If you would like to share the story of your exam success or if you have any questions or comments in regard to our products, please contact us at **800-673-8175** or **support@mometrix.com**.

Thanks again for your business and we wish you continued success!

Sincerely,
The Mometrix Test Preparation Team

TABLE OF CONTENTS

Introduction

Thank you for purchasing this resource! You have made the choice to prepare yourself for a test that could have a huge impact on your future, and this guide is designed to help you be fully ready for test day. Obviously, it's important to have a solid understanding of the test material, but you also need to be prepared for the unique environment and stressors of the test, so that you can perform to the best of your abilities.

For this purpose, the first section that appears in this guide is the **Secret Keys**. We've devoted countless hours to meticulously researching what works and what doesn't, and we've boiled down our findings to the five most impactful steps you can take to improve your performance on the test. We start at the beginning with study planning and move through the preparation process, all the way to the testing strategies that will help you get the most out of what you know when you're finally sitting in front of the test.

We recommend that you start preparing for your test as far in advance as possible. However, if you've bought this guide as a last-minute study resource and only have a few days before your test, we recommend that you skip over the first two Secret Keys since they address a long-term study plan.

If you struggle with **test anxiety**, we strongly encourage you to check out our recommendations for how you can overcome it. Test anxiety is a formidable foe, but it can be beaten, and we want to make sure you have the tools you need to defeat it.

Secret Key #1 – Plan Big, Study Small

There's a lot riding on your performance. If you want to ace this test, you're going to need to keep your skills sharp and the material fresh in your mind. You need a plan that lets you review everything you need to know while still fitting in your schedule. We'll break this strategy down into three categories.

Information Organization

Start with the information you already have: the official test outline. From this, you can make a complete list of all the concepts you need to cover before the test. Organize these concepts into groups that can be studied together, and create a list of any related vocabulary you need to learn so you can brush up on any difficult terms. You'll want to keep this vocabulary list handy once you actually start studying since you may need to add to it along the way.

Time Management

Once you have your set of study concepts, decide how to spread them out over the time you have left before the test. Break your study plan into small, clear goals so you have a manageable task for each day and know exactly what you're doing. Then just focus on one small step at a time. When you manage your time this way, you don't need to spend hours at a time studying. Studying a small block of content for a short period each day helps you retain information better and avoid stressing over how much you have left to do. You can relax knowing that you have a plan to cover everything in time. In order for this strategy to be effective though, you have to start studying early and stick to your schedule. Avoid the exhaustion and futility that comes from last-minute cramming!

Study Environment

The environment you study in has a big impact on your learning. Studying in a coffee shop, while probably more enjoyable, is not likely to be as fruitful as studying in a quiet room. It's important to keep distractions to a minimum. You're only planning to study for a short block of time, so make the most of it. Don't pause to check your phone or get up to find a snack. It's also important to **avoid multitasking**. Research has consistently shown that multitasking will make your studying dramatically less effective. Your study area should also be comfortable and well-lit so you don't have the distraction of straining your eyes or sitting on an uncomfortable chair.

The time of day you study is also important. You want to be rested and alert. Don't wait until just before bedtime. Study when you'll be most likely to comprehend and remember. Even better, if you know what time of day your test will be, set that time aside for study. That way your brain will be used to working on that subject at that specific time and you'll have a better chance of recalling information.

Finally, it can be helpful to team up with others who are studying for the same test. Your actual studying should be done in as isolated an environment as possible, but the work of organizing the information and setting up the study plan can be divided up. In between study sessions, you can discuss with your teammates the concepts that you're all studying and quiz each other on the details. Just be sure that your teammates are as serious about the test as you are. If you find that your study time is being replaced with social time, you might need to find a new team.

Secret Key #2 – Make Your Studying Count

You're devoting a lot of time and effort to preparing for this test, so you want to be absolutely certain it will pay off. This means doing more than just reading the content and hoping you can remember it on test day. It's important to make every minute of study count. There are two main areas you can focus on to make your studying count:

Retention

It doesn't matter how much time you study if you can't remember the material. You need to make sure you are retaining the concepts. To check your retention of the information you're learning, try recalling it at later times with minimal prompting. Try carrying around flashcards and glance at one or two from time to time or ask a friend who's also studying for the test to quiz you.

To enhance your retention, look for ways to put the information into practice so that you can apply it rather than simply recalling it. If you're using the information in practical ways, it will be much easier to remember. Similarly, it helps to solidify a concept in your mind if you're not only reading it to yourself but also explaining it to someone else. Ask a friend to let you teach them about a concept you're a little shaky on (or speak aloud to an imaginary audience if necessary). As you try to summarize, define, give examples, and answer your friend's questions, you'll understand the concepts better and they will stay with you longer. Finally, step back for a big picture view and ask yourself how each piece of information fits with the whole subject. When you link the different concepts together and see them working together as a whole, it's easier to remember the individual components.

Finally, practice showing your work on any multi-step problems, even if you're just studying. Writing out each step you take to solve a problem will help solidify the process in your mind, and you'll be more likely to remember it during the test.

Modality

Modality simply refers to the means or method by which you study. Choosing a study modality that fits your own individual learning style is crucial. No two people learn best in exactly the same way, so it's important to know your strengths and use them to your advantage.

For example, if you learn best by visualization, focus on visualizing a concept in your mind and draw an image or a diagram. Try color-coding your notes, illustrating them, or creating symbols that will trigger your mind to recall a learned concept. If you learn best by hearing or discussing information, find a study partner who learns the same way or read aloud to yourself. Think about how to put the information in your own words. Imagine that you are giving a lecture on the topic and record yourself so you can listen to it later.

For any learning style, flashcards can be helpful. Organize the information so you can take advantage of spare moments to review. Underline key words or phrases. Use different colors for different categories. Mnemonic devices (such as creating a short list in which every item starts with the same letter) can also help with retention. Find what works best for you and use it to store the information in your mind most effectively and easily.

Secret Key #3 – Practice the Right Way

Your success on test day depends not only on how many hours you put into preparing, but also on whether you prepared the right way. It's good to check along the way to see if your studying is paying off. One of the most effective ways to do this is by taking practice tests to evaluate your progress. Practice tests are useful because they show exactly where you need to improve. Every time you take a practice test, pay special attention to these three groups of questions:

- The questions you got wrong
- The questions you had to guess on, even if you guessed right
- The questions you found difficult or slow to work through

This will show you exactly what your weak areas are, and where you need to devote more study time. Ask yourself why each of these questions gave you trouble. Was it because you didn't understand the material? Was it because you didn't remember the vocabulary? Do you need more repetitions on this type of question to build speed and confidence? Dig into those questions and figure out how you can strengthen your weak areas as you go back to review the material.

Additionally, many practice tests have a section explaining the answer choices. It can be tempting to read the explanation and think that you now have a good understanding of the concept. However, an explanation likely only covers part of the question's broader context. Even if the explanation makes sense, **go back and investigate** every concept related to the question until you're positive you have a thorough understanding.

As you go along, keep in mind that the practice test is just that: practice. Memorizing these questions and answers will not be very helpful on the actual test because it is unlikely to have any of the same exact questions. If you only know the right answers to the sample questions, you won't be prepared for the real thing. **Study the concepts** until you understand them fully, and then you'll be able to answer any question that shows up on the test.

It's important to wait on the practice tests until you're ready. If you take a test on your first day of study, you may be overwhelmed by the amount of material covered and how much you need to learn. Work up to it gradually.

On test day, you'll need to be prepared for answering questions, managing your time, and using the test-taking strategies you've learned. It's a lot to balance, like a mental marathon that will have a big impact on your future. Like training for a marathon, you'll need to start slowly and work your way up. When test day arrives, you'll be ready.

Start with the strategies you've read in the first two Secret Keys—plan your course and study in the way that works best for you. If you have time, consider using multiple study resources to get different approaches to the same concepts. It can be helpful to see difficult concepts from more than one angle. Then find a good source for practice tests. Many times, the test website will suggest potential study resources or provide sample tests.

Practice Test Strategy

When you're ready to start taking practice tests, follow this strategy:

1. Take the first test with no time constraints and with your notes and study guide handy. Take your time and focus on applying the strategies you've learned.
2. Take the second practice test open-book as well, but set a timer and practice pacing yourself to finish in time.
3. Take any other practice tests as if it were test day. Set a timer and put away your study materials. Sit at a table or desk in a quiet room, imagine yourself at the testing center, and answer questions as quickly and accurately as possible.
4. Keep repeating step 3 on a regular basis until you run out of practice tests or it's time for the actual test. Your mind will be ready for the schedule and stress of test day, and you'll be able to focus on recalling the material you've learned.

Secret Key #4 – Pace Yourself

Once you're fully prepared for the material on the test, your biggest challenge on test day will be managing your time. Just knowing that the clock is ticking can make you panic even if you have plenty of time left. Work on pacing yourself so you can build confidence against the time constraints of the exam. Pacing is a difficult skill to master, especially in a high-pressure environment, so **practice is vital**.

Set time expectations for your pace based on how much time is available. For example, if a section has 60 questions and the time limit is 30 minutes, you know you have to average 30 seconds or less per question in order to answer them all. Although 30 seconds is the hard limit, set 25 seconds per question as your goal, so you reserve extra time to spend on harder questions. When you budget extra time for the harder questions, you no longer have any reason to stress when those questions take longer to answer.

Don't let this time expectation distract you from working through the test at a calm, steady pace, but keep it in mind so you don't spend too much time on any one question. Recognize that taking extra time on one question you don't understand may keep you from answering two that you do understand later in the test. If your time limit for a question is up and you're still not sure of the answer, mark it and move on, and come back to it later if the time and the test format allow. If the testing format doesn't allow you to return to earlier questions, just make an educated guess; then put it out of your mind and move on.

On the easier questions, be careful not to rush. It may seem wise to hurry through them so you have more time for the challenging ones, but it's not worth missing one if you know the concept and just didn't take the time to read the question fully. Work efficiently but make sure you understand the question and have looked at all of the answer choices, since more than one may seem right at first.

Even if you're paying attention to the time, you may find yourself a little behind at some point. You should speed up to get back on track, but do so wisely. Don't panic; just take a few seconds less on each question until you're caught up. Don't guess without thinking, but do look through the answer choices and eliminate any you know are wrong. If you can get down to two choices, it is often worthwhile to guess from those. Once you've chosen an answer, move on and don't dwell on any that you skipped or had to hurry through. If a question was taking too long, chances are it was one of the harder ones, so you weren't as likely to get it right anyway.

On the other hand, if you find yourself getting ahead of schedule, it may be beneficial to slow down a little. The more quickly you work, the more likely you are to make a careless mistake that will affect your score. You've budgeted time for each question, so don't be afraid to spend that time. Practice an efficient but careful pace to get the most out of the time you have.

Secret Key #5 – Have a Plan for Guessing

When you're taking the test, you may find yourself stuck on a question. Some of the answer choices seem better than others, but you don't see the one answer choice that is obviously correct. What do you do?

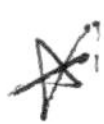

The scenario described above is very common, yet most test takers have not effectively prepared for it. Developing and practicing a plan for guessing may be one of the single most effective uses of your time as you get ready for the exam.

In developing your plan for guessing, there are three questions to address:

- When should you start the guessing process?
- How should you narrow down the choices?
- Which answer should you choose?

When to Start the Guessing Process

Unless your plan for guessing is to select C every time (which, despite its merits, is not what we recommend), you need to leave yourself enough time to apply your answer elimination strategies. Since you have a limited amount of time for each question, that means that if you're going to give yourself the best shot at guessing correctly, you have to decide quickly whether or not you will guess.

Of course, the best-case scenario is that you don't have to guess at all, so first, see if you can answer the question based on your knowledge of the subject and basic reasoning skills. Focus on the key words in the question and try to jog your memory of related topics. Give yourself a chance to bring the knowledge to mind, but once you realize that you don't have (or you can't access) the knowledge you need to answer the question, it's time to start the guessing process.

It's almost always better to start the guessing process too early than too late. It only takes a few seconds to remember something and answer the question from knowledge. Carefully eliminating wrong answer choices takes longer. Plus, going through the process of eliminating answer choices can actually help jog your memory.

Summary: Start the guessing process as soon as you decide that you can't answer the question based on your knowledge.

How to Narrow Down the Choices

The next chapter in this book (**Test-Taking Strategies**) includes a wide range of strategies for how to approach questions and how to look for answer choices to eliminate. You will definitely want to read those carefully, practice them, and figure out which ones work best for you. Here though, we're going to address a mindset rather than a particular strategy.

Your chances of guessing an answer correctly depend on how many options you are choosing from.

How many choices you have	How likely you are to guess correctly
5	20%
4	25%
3	33%
2	50%
1	100%

You can see from this chart just how valuable it is to be able to eliminate incorrect answers and make an educated guess, but there are two things that many test takers do that cause them to miss out on the benefits of guessing:

- Accidentally eliminating the correct answer
- Selecting an answer based on an impression

We'll look at the first one here, and the second one in the next section.

To avoid accidentally eliminating the correct answer, we recommend a thought exercise called **the $5 challenge**. In this challenge, you only eliminate an answer choice from contention if you are willing to bet $5 on it being wrong. Why $5? Five dollars is a small but not insignificant amount of money. It's an amount you could afford to lose but wouldn't want to throw away. And while losing $5 once might not hurt too much, doing it twenty times will set you back $100. In the same way, each small decision you make—eliminating a choice here, guessing on a question there—won't by itself impact your score very much, but when you put them all together, they can make a big difference. By holding each answer choice elimination decision to a higher standard, you can reduce the risk of accidentally eliminating the correct answer.

The $5 challenge can also be applied in a positive sense: If you are willing to bet $5 that an answer choice *is* correct, go ahead and mark it as correct.

Summary: Only eliminate an answer choice if you are willing to bet $5 that it is wrong.

Which Answer to Choose

You're taking the test. You've run into a hard question and decided you'll have to guess. You've eliminated all the answer choices you're willing to bet $5 on. Now you have to pick an answer. Why do we even need to talk about this? Why can't you just pick whichever one you feel like when the time comes?

The answer to these questions is that if you don't come into the test with a plan, you'll rely on your impression to select an answer choice, and if you do that, you risk falling into a trap. The test writers know that everyone who takes their test will be guessing on some of the questions, so they intentionally write wrong answer choices to seem plausible. You still have to pick an answer though, and if the wrong answer choices are designed to look right, how can you ever be sure that you're not falling for their trap? The best solution we've found to this dilemma is to take the decision out of your hands entirely. Here is the process we recommend:

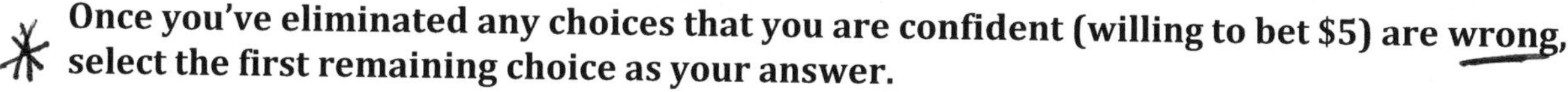

Once you've eliminated any choices that you are confident (willing to bet $5) are wrong, select the first remaining choice as your answer.

Whether you choose to select the first remaining choice, the second, or the last, the important thing is that you use some preselected standard. Using this approach guarantees that you will not be enticed into selecting an answer choice that looks right, because you are not basing your decision on how the answer choices look.

This is not meant to make you question your knowledge. Instead, it is to help you recognize the difference between your knowledge and your impressions. There's a huge difference between thinking an answer is right because of what you know, and thinking an answer is right because it looks or sounds like it should be right.

Summary: To ensure that your selection is appropriately random, make a predetermined selection from among all answer choices you have not eliminated.

Test-Taking Strategies

This section contains a list of test-taking strategies that you may find helpful as you work through the test. By taking what you know and applying logical thought, you can maximize your chances of answering any question correctly!

It is very important to realize that every question is different and every person is different: no single strategy will work on every question, and no single strategy will work for every person. That's why we've included all of them here, so you can try them out and determine which ones work best for different types of questions and which ones work best for you.

Question Strategies

Read Carefully

Read the question and answer choices carefully. Don't miss the question because you misread the terms. You have plenty of time to read each question thoroughly and make sure you understand what is being asked. Yet a happy medium must be attained, so don't waste too much time. You must read carefully, but efficiently.

Contextual Clues

Look for contextual clues. If the question includes a word you are not familiar with, look at the immediate context for some indication of what the word might mean. Contextual clues can often give you all the information you need to decipher the meaning of an unfamiliar word. Even if you can't determine the meaning, you may be able to narrow down the possibilities enough to make a solid guess at the answer to the question.

Prefixes

If you're having trouble with a word in the question or answer choices, try dissecting it. Take advantage of every clue that the word might include. Prefixes and suffixes can be a huge help. Usually they allow you to determine a basic meaning. Pre- means before, post- means after, pro - is positive, de- is negative. From prefixes and suffixes, you can get an idea of the general meaning of the word and try to put it into context.

Hedge Words

Watch out for critical hedge words, such as *likely, may, can, sometimes, often, almost, mostly, usually, generally, rarely*, and *sometimes*. Question writers insert these hedge phrases to cover every possibility. Often an answer choice will be wrong simply because it leaves no room for exception. Be on guard for answer choices that have definitive words such as *exactly* and *always*.

Switchback Words

Stay alert for *switchbacks*. These are the words and phrases frequently used to alert you to shifts in thought. The most common switchback words are *but, although*, and *however*. Others include *nevertheless, on the other hand, even though, while, in spite of, despite, regardless of*. Switchback words are important to catch because they can change the direction of the question or an answer choice.

FACE VALUE

When in doubt, use common sense. Accept the situation in the problem at face value. Don't read too much into it. These problems will not require you to make wild assumptions. If you have to go beyond creativity and warp time or space in order to have an answer choice fit the question, then you should move on and consider the other answer choices. These are normal problems rooted in reality. The applicable relationship or explanation may not be readily apparent, but it is there for you to figure out. Use your common sense to interpret anything that isn't clear.

Answer Choice Strategies

ANSWER SELECTION

The most thorough way to pick an answer choice is to identify and eliminate wrong answers until only one is left, then confirm it is the correct answer. Sometimes an answer choice may immediately seem right, but be careful. The test writers will usually put more than one reasonable answer choice on each question, so take a second to read all of them and make sure that the other choices are not equally obvious. As long as you have time left, it is better to read every answer choice than to pick the first one that looks right without checking the others.

ANSWER CHOICE FAMILIES

An answer choice family consists of two (in rare cases, three) answer choices that are very similar in construction and cannot all be true at the same time. If you see two answer choices that are direct opposites or parallels, one of them is usually the correct answer. For instance, if one answer choice says that quantity *x* increases and another either says that quantity *x* decreases (opposite) or says that quantity *y* increases (parallel), then those answer choices would fall into the same family. An answer choice that doesn't match the construction of the answer choice family is more likely to be incorrect. Most questions will not have answer choice families, but when they do appear, you should be prepared to recognize them.

ELIMINATE ANSWERS

Eliminate answer choices as soon as you realize they are wrong, but make sure you consider all possibilities. If you are eliminating answer choices and realize that the last one you are left with is also wrong, don't panic. Start over and consider each choice again. There may be something you missed the first time that you will realize on the second pass.

AVOID FACT TRAPS

Don't be distracted by an answer choice that is factually true but doesn't answer the question. You are looking for the choice that answers the question. Stay focused on what the question is asking for so you don't accidentally pick an answer that is true but incorrect. Always go back to the question and make sure the answer choice you've selected actually answers the question and is not merely a true statement.

EXTREME STATEMENTS

In general, you should avoid answers that put forth extreme actions as standard practice or proclaim controversial ideas as established fact. An answer choice that states the "process should be used in certain situations, if..." is much more likely to be correct than one that states the "process should be discontinued completely." The first is a calm rational statement and doesn't even make a definitive, uncompromising stance, using a hedge word *if* to provide wiggle room, whereas the second choice is a radical idea and far more extreme.

- **BENCHMARK**

  As you read through the answer choices and you come across one that seems to answer the question well, mentally select that answer choice. This is not your final answer, but it's the one that will help you evaluate the other answer choices. The one that you selected is your benchmark or standard for judging each of the other answer choices. Every other answer choice must be compared to your benchmark. That choice is correct until proven otherwise by another answer choice beating it. If you find a better answer, then that one becomes your new benchmark. Once you've decided that no other choice answers the question as well as your benchmark, you have your final answer.

PREDICT THE ANSWER

Before you even start looking at the answer choices, it is often best to try to predict the answer. When you come up with the answer on your own, it is easier to avoid distractions and traps because you will know exactly what to look for. The right answer choice is unlikely to be word-for-word what you came up with, but it should be a close match. Even if you are confident that you have the right answer, you should still take the time to read each option before moving on.

General Strategies

TOUGH QUESTIONS

If you are stumped on a problem or it appears too hard or too difficult, don't waste time. Move on! Remember though, if you can quickly check for obviously incorrect answer choices, your chances of guessing correctly are greatly improved. Before you completely give up, at least try to knock out a couple of possible answers. Eliminate what you can and then guess at the remaining answer choices before moving on.

CHECK YOUR WORK

Since you will probably not know every term listed and the answer to every question, it is important that you get credit for the ones that you do know. Don't miss any questions through careless mistakes. If at all possible, try to take a second to look back over your answer selection and make sure you've selected the correct answer choice and haven't made a costly careless mistake (such as marking an answer choice that you didn't mean to mark). This quick double check should more than pay for itself in caught mistakes for the time it costs.

PACE YOURSELF

It's easy to be overwhelmed when you're looking at a page full of questions; your mind is confused and full of random thoughts, and the clock is ticking down faster than you would like. Calm down and maintain the pace that you have set for yourself. Especially as you get down to the last few minutes of the test, don't let the small numbers on the clock make you panic. As long as you are on track by monitoring your pace, you are guaranteed to have time for each question.

DON'T RUSH

It is very easy to make errors when you are in a hurry. Maintaining a fast pace in answering questions is pointless if it makes you miss questions that you would have gotten right otherwise. Test writers like to include distracting information and wrong answers that seem right. Taking a little extra time to avoid careless mistakes can make all the difference in your test score. Find a pace that allows you to be confident in the answers that you select.

Keep Moving

Panicking will not help you pass the test, so do your best to stay calm and keep moving. Taking deep breaths and going through the answer elimination steps you practiced can help to break through a stress barrier and keep your pace.

Final Notes

The combination of a solid foundation of content knowledge and the confidence that comes from practicing your plan for applying that knowledge is the key to maximizing your performance on test day. As your foundation of content knowledge is built up and strengthened, you'll find that the strategies included in this chapter become more and more effective in helping you quickly sift through the distractions and traps of the test to isolate the correct answer.

Now it's time to move on to the test content chapters of this book, but be sure to keep your goal in mind. As you read, think about how you will be able to apply this information on the test. If you've already seen sample questions for the test and you have an idea of the question format and style, try to come up with questions of your own that you can answer based on what you're reading. This will give you valuable practice applying your knowledge in the same ways you can expect to on test day.

Good luck and good studying!

Pharmacology for Technicians

Patient's Medical History

A patient's medical history may include the following information:

- Medications taken by the patient, including OTC and dietary supplements
- Chronic medical conditions
- Acute medical conditions
- Patterns of prescription compliance
- Allergies to substances, including medications and food
- Any interactions that may occur, including drug-drug, drug-food, and so forth

Knowing a patient's medical history allows the pharmacist to determine any potential **risk** to the patient. For example, some medical conditions may contraindicate the use of certain medications. An allergy to a certain medication may indicate a potential allergy to other medications within that class. Many medications are known to interact with others. If the pharmacist is aware of the patient's medication history, a **drug interaction**, which can have serious consequences, can be prevented.

OTC Medications and Dietary Supplements

OTC medications – Medications available "**over the counter**," i.e. without a prescription. The FDA regulates both the sale and manufacture of OTC medications as per the Federal Food, Drug, and Cosmetic Act. Some medications are classified as over the counter, but because of federal or local laws, are only available for sale by a qualified pharmacy employee after the patient receives counseling or signs a ledger (for example, medications containing pseudoephedrine or emergency contraceptives). Local laws may cause a medication to be OTC in one part of the country and only available by prescription in other areas.

Dietary supplements – Unlike OTC medications, dietary supplements are not regulated by the FDA. The **Dietary Health and Supplement Act of 1994** identifies dietary supplements as any product that meets the following guidelines:

- Contains a vitamin, mineral, herb, botanical, and/or amino acid
- Marketed as a capsule, tablet, powder or liquid
- Not intended to be the sole source of nutrition
- Contains the labeling "dietary supplement"

OTC Medications Ingredients

Many over the counter preparations contain combinations of different **ingredients**, especially medications intended to treat coughs and colds or the flu. When purchasing over the counter medications (or selling them), it is important to double-check the ingredients to be sure that medications are not being **duplicated**. For example, the medications Theraflu and Nyquil both contain acetaminophen and dextromethorphan – two medications that can be dangerous if overdosed. Additionally, over the counter sleep aids frequently contain the same ingredients found in antihistamines. Migraine formulas frequently contain caffeine, which can cause sleeplessness and a jittery sensation when too much is consumed. If you are selling medications and notice a potential doubling of active ingredients, notify a pharmacist so he or she can counsel the patient.

Chronic Conditions Verses Acute Conditions

Chronic conditions may develop slowly, over time, and are persistent. They may go into remission and then recur. A chronic condition can be mild, serious or fatal in nature. Chronic conditions may require long-term medical treatment, which may focus on symptom relief rather than cure. Examples of chronic conditions include heart disease, diabetes, and cancer.

Acute conditions may develop suddenly and resolve quickly. Symptoms may be intense. Like a chronic condition, an acute condition may be mild, severe, or fatal. Examples of acute conditions include strep throat, pneumonia, and gastritis.

Compliance

Compliant patients are conscientious about following the recommendations given by their medical providers. They take medications as directed and follow up with necessary tests and procedures. Examples of **noncompliance** include:

- Taking less of the medication than was prescribed
- Stopping medication early
- Taking medication at the wrong time of day
- Using expired medications

Failure to take a medication as directed may cause the medication not to work as intended or could create unwanted effects. A number of factors, including physical issues, cognitive problems, fear of side effects, and misunderstandings, can cause noncompliance. Many pharmacies have developed **systems** to help patients be more compliant, including automating refills; reminder phone calls, texts, and emails; and notifications to doctors when patients are noncompliant.

Medication Allergy

Symptoms indicating an **allergy** to a medication include the following:

- Skin reactions, including redness and rashes
- Hives
- Swelling, which may occur in the face, throat, tongue, or other areas of the body
- Difficulty breathing, wheezing, or chest tightness
- Rapid heartbeat or irregular heartbeat

If these reactions are severe, they may indicate an **anaphylactic reaction**. Anaphylaxis is life threatening and requires immediate emergency treatment. If someone is suspected of having an anaphylactic reaction to any substance, call 911 immediately. Patients often confuse adverse effects with allergic reactions. When a patient states that they have an allergic reaction to a medication, ask about the symptoms the patient experiences in order to classify the reaction correctly.

Food or Medication Allergy History

Some medications and supplements that might be prescribed to a patient contain **food-based ingredients**. For example, the coatings of medications may contain a number of incipient ingredients such as lactose, maltodextrin, and other starches that could elicit an allergic reaction in a person who is sensitive to those ingredients. Some medications, including the hormone medication Prometrium and a number of prescription creams contain peanut oil. A person with a seafood allergy may need to avoid certain omega-3 supplements, and some calcium products that are derived from shellfish. Patients who are vegan will not wish to take capsules made from gelatin while patients with celiac disease or gluten intolerance should avoid medications made with gluten fillers. When in doubt, contact the manufacturer.

Drug Interactions

- **Drug-drug interactions** occur when the ingredients of one drug affect the ingredients of another drug. They may cause the other drug to not absorb properly, may negate the effect of the drug, or may enhance the action of the drug. In some cases, drug manufacturers have taken advantage of this interaction and combined two medications that are more effective taken together than when taken individually.
- **Drug-food interactions** occur when certain foods effect the action of a medication. Some foods may impair the absorption of a medication, while other foods may bind to the medication and change its action. Some medications should be taken with food while it is recommended that others be taken on an empty stomach.
- **Drug-condition interactions** occur when a patient's condition affects how a medication works, or when the medication could worsen the patient's condition. For example, certain nasal decongestants can be dangerous for people with high blood pressure, and people with a blood-clotting disorder should avoid blood thinners like aspirin and warfarin.

Adverse Drug Reactions

An adverse drug reaction is an undesired reaction that occurs when a medication is taken in a manner consistent with its standard dosing. An adverse drug reaction may occur the first time a medication is taken, or it may develop over time. Adverse drug reactions may be **local** or **systemic**. Serious adverse drug reactions require **intervention** to prevent permanent damage or impairment and may result in hospitalization or death. The different types of reactions that may occur are:

- Augmented pharmacologic effects including intolerance and side effects
- Idiosyncratic and unpredictable effects
- Chronic effects
- Delayed effects
- End of treatment effects
- Therapy failure
- Genetic reactions

Polypharmacy

Polypharmacy occurs when a patient is taking multiple medications, especially if the patient is taking more medications than are actually necessary to treat their condition. This situation is most common in the elderly population and in people who are treating multiple medical conditions, although it can also occur in the general population. One of the most common problems with polypharmacy is the risk of **serious drug interactions**. Additionally, numerous drug side effects may occur. Polypharmacy often occurs when a patient is seeing multiple doctors to treat different conditions, and each doctor is not aware of what the other doctors are prescribing. Pharmacy technicians can help prevent polypharmacy by informing the pharmacist of **medication interactions** and **multiple medications** from different doctors. Pharmacists can help by conferring with the patient's doctors to make sure each one knows what the other has prescribed and reviewing the medications with the patient and/or caregiver.

Routes of Administration

Medications may be administered through a variety of **routes**. Some of the most common are:

- **Orally**, or by mouth, such as with oral tablets, capsules, elixirs and suspensions
- **Nasally**, or by nose, such as nasal sprays or drips
- **Intravenously**, or through the veins
- **Intramuscularly**, or into the muscle
- **Subcutaneous**, or under the skin
- **Epidural**, or infusion into the epidural space
- **Transdermal**, or absorbed through the skin, such as patches and creams
- **Rectally**, or through the anus, such as suppositories and some creams
- **Sublingual**, or under the tongue
- **Inhalation**, or inhaled into the lungs, such as many sprays and nebulized solutions
- **Ocular**, or into the eye, such as many solutions and suspensions
- **Aurally**, or into the ear, such as many solutions and suspensions

Tablet, Capsule, Elixir, and Suspension

The **tablet** is the most common oral dosage form. It may be composed of powder firmly compressed into the tablet shape and may be coated to prevent a foul taste or to delay release of the medication. Tablets can also be more complex in nature, using delayed release systems such as the osmotic release system. **Capsules** use a hard or soft gelling agent coating to encapsulate pellets, powder, or liquid ingredients. Many capsules are made of gelatin, an animal derived product, while others are made of plant-based polysaccharides. An **elixir** is a liquid solution. The active ingredients are dissolved into the liquid carrier. Solutions do not require shaking to mix the ingredients. A **suspension** consists of medication that is suspended in a liquid carrier. Some suspensions require mixing with distilled water before transfer to the patient. Suspensions require shaking before dosing, as the ingredients may settle.

IV Admixture

IV admixture is a type of compounding in which a drug is added to a 50 mL or larger container of fluid to be administered intravenously. Proper IV admixture requires skill and finesse, as it is crucial to deliver the proper amount of medication to the patient, with no room for error. Knowledge of proper **aseptic technique** is required for successful IV admixture. Failure to adhere to proper technique could result in overdosing or under dosing the patient or introducing dangerous microbes or other contaminants into the patient's system.

Drawing a Drug from an Ampule

When using a medication that is stored in an **ampule**, special precautions must be taken to prevent injury when opening the ampule and to keep particulates such as chips of paint and glass from being introduced into the medication.

1. Flick or tap the top of the ampule to remove any medication from the tip.
2. Wipe the top of the ampule with an alcohol swab.
3. Wrap the tip with gauze and quickly snap the tip off, away from the body and face.
4. Using a syringe fitted with a filter needle, withdraw the exact amount of medication, being careful to keep the needle from touching the edges of the ampule.
5. Ampule may be tipped slightly in order to withdraw all the medication.

6. Before injecting the medication, the filter needle must be removed, and a sterile regular needle must be attached.
7. Dispose of the filter needle and both pieces of the ampule in the sharps container

Pharmacokinetics

Pharmacokinetics is the process of how medication is metabolized by the body. Knowledge of the pharmacokinetics of any medication is required to determine the rate at which a medication will be metabolized and eliminated by the patient. Pharmacokinetics is broken down into four different stages: **absorption**, **distribution**, **metabolization**, and **elimination**. Because every patient is different, different factors will have an effect on the rate, making it difficult to predict exactly how any medication will be absorbed in any one patient. Some of the factors affecting the rate of metabolism include:

- Patient's age
- Recent food, drink or alcohol consumption
- The effect of other medications that have been taken

"Half-Life"

During a given unit of time, a portion of the drug will be metabolized and eliminated by the body. During each **half-life period**, half of the medication concentrated in the blood will be metabolized and eliminated. Although medications may be in the same class, the effects of one may last longer than the effects of others. This is due in part to the medications' half-lives. A medication with a half-life of 14 hours will eliminate half of the blood concentration of the medication in every 14-hour increment, while a medication with a half-life of 5 hours will eliminate half the blood concentration of the medication in each 5-hour increment. This means that the medication with the 5-hour half-life will be out of the system much faster. Medication half-life determines the **dosage rate**. The 5-hour half-life medication may require twice daily dosing, while the 14-hour half-life medication requires once daily dosing.

Zero Order Kinetics

In zero order kinetics, a substance is processed at a steady rate by your body, regardless of the concentration of the substance in your blood. Alcohol is typically processed by the body in zero kinetic fashion. For example, if your body can process 1 ounce of alcohol every hour, effectively eliminating it from your system, but you drink 3 ounces of alcohol in one hour, your body will continue to process the alcohol at a rate of 1 ounce per hour. After one hour, your body will have processed 1 ounce of alcohol, after two hours, your body will have processed the second ounce of alcohol, and at three hours, your body will have processed the third ounce of alcohol. If you did not drink any more alcohol after those 3 ounces, you will no longer have alcohol in your system.

Age of Person Affect Response of Medication

The very young and the very old frequently respond differently to medication. They may have a higher or lower than anticipated **response** to the strength, they may experience unusual **effects**, or a dose that seems correct when calculated by weight may prove to be an **overdose**. Many medications have not been approved by the FDA for use in children but are used "off label." Many medications have not been studied in pediatric or geriatric populations, and unexpected reactions may occur. If a medication is prescribed by a physician that is not approved for use in either of these populations, notify the pharmacist, who will use his or her own professional judgment as to whether to dispense the medication or notify the physician.

Abbreviations

When a Medication Should Be Taken

Abbreviation	Meaning
ac	before meals
bid	twice daily
hs	at bedtime
pc	after meals
prn	as needed
q4h/q4°	every 4 hours
qd	daily
qid	four times daily
qod	every other day
tid	three times daily

Drug Dosage

Abbreviation	Meaning
cap	capsule
gtt	drop
i, ii, iii, iv	1, 2, 3, 4 (Roman numerals are often used to identify quantities on prescriptions)
mcg/μg	microgram (μg is not being used as much because when written out, it is often mistaken for mg. If unsure, confirm dose with prescriber.)
mg	milligrams
mL	milliliter
ss	one-half
tab	tablet
tbsp.	tablespoon (15 ml)
tsp.	teaspoon (5 ml)

Route of Administration

Abbreviation	Meaning
ad	right ear
as	left ear
au	both ears
c	with
od	right eye
os	left eye
ou	both eyes
po	by mouth
sl	sublingual
top	topically

Sample Sigs

Sigs	Understandable dosing instructions
i tab po bid prn	Take one tablet by mouth twice daily as needed.
ii gtts au tid	Instill two drops in both ears three times daily.
i – ii tabs q4-6h prn pain	Take one to two tablets every four to six hours as needed for pain.
apply top qd	Apply topically once daily.
i – ii tsp po tid ac	Take one to two teaspoons by mouth three times daily before meals.
5 – 10 mL po q8h prn cough	Take 5 to 10 mL by mouth every eight hours as needed for cough. (Alternately, take 1 to 2 teaspoons by mouth every eight hours as needed for cough.)
Inj 3 units sq pc	Inject 3 units subcutaneously after meals.
i gtt os q2°	Instill one drop in the left eye every two hours.
ii cap po qhs	Take two capsules by mouth every night at bedtime.
i tab qam, may repeat x1 prn	Take one tablet every morning. May repeat once

Drug Abbreviation

Many medications are identified with common abbreviations. These are some of the most common:

Common Abbreviation	Medication
APAP	acetaminophen
ASA	aspirin
Fe	iron
HCTZ	hydrochlorothiazide
INH	isoniazid
MgSO4	magnesium sulfate
MOM	milk of magnesia
MVI	multivitamin
NS	normal saline
NTG	nitroglycerin
PCN	penicillin
PNV	prenatal vitamins
SMZ/TMP	sulfamethoxazole/ trimethoprim
TAC	triamcinolone
TCN	tetracycline

Medication Generic Name

Brand Name	Generic Name
Abilify	aripiprazole
AcipHex	rabeprazole
Actonel	risedronate
Actos	pioglitazone
Adderall	dextroamphetamine/amphetamine
Advair	fluticasone/salmeterol
Allegra	fexofenadine
Alphagan	brimonidine

Brand Name	Generic Name
Altace	ramipril
Ambien	zolpidem
Amoxil	amoxicillin
Aricept	donepezil
Astelin	azelastine
Atacand	candesartan
Avalide	irbesartan/hydrochlorothiazide
Avapro	irbesartan
Avelox	moxifloxacin
Benicar	olmesartan
Biaxin	clarithromycin
Boniva	ibandronate
Byetta	exenatide
Celebrex	celecoxib
Cialis	tadalafil
Ciprodex	ciprofloxacin/dexamethasone
Combivent	albuterol/ipratropium
Concerta	methylphenidate
Coreg	carvedilol
Cosopt	dorzolamide/timolol
Coumadin	warfarin
Cozaar	losartan
Crestor	rosuvastatin
Cymbalta	duloxetine
Depakote	divalproex
Detrol	tolterodine
Digitek	digoxin
Dilantin	phenytoin
Diovan	valsartan
Effexor	venlafaxine
Evista	raloxifene
Flomax	tamsulosin
Flonase	fluticasone
Flovent	fluticasone
Fosamax	alendronate
Geodon	ziprasidone
Glucophage	metformin
Humalog	insulin lispro
Hyzaar	hydrochlorothiazide/losartan
Imitrex	sumatriptan
Inderal	propranolol
Keppra	levetiracetam
Klor-Con	potassium
Lamisil	terbinafine
Lanoxin	digoxin
Lantus	insulin glargine
Levaquin	levofloxacin

Brand Name	Generic Name
Levitra	vardenafil
Levoxyl	levothyroxine
Lexapro	escitalopram
Lidoderm	lidocaine
Lipitor	atorvastatin
Lotrel	amlodipine/ benazepril
Lumigan	bimatoprost
Lunesta	eszopiclone
Lyrica	pregabalin
Micardis	telmisartan
Mobic	meloxicam
Namenda	memantine
Nasonex	mometasone
Nexium	esomeprazole
Norvasc	amlodipine
Omnicef	cefdinir
Patanol	olopatadine
Paxil	paroxetine
Percocet	oxycodone/acetaminophen
Plavix	clopidogrel
Pravachol	pravastatin
Premarin	conjugated estrogens
Prevacid	lansoprazole
Prilosec	omeprazole
Protonix	pantoprazole
Provigil	modafinil
Pulmicort	budesonide
Requip	ropinirole
Rhinocort	budesonide
Risperdal	risperidone
Ritalin	methylphenidate
Seroquel	quetiapine
Singulair	montelukast
Skelaxin	metaxalone
Spiriva	tiotropium
Strattera	atomoxetine
Synthroid	levothyroxine
TobraDex	tobramycin/dexamethasone
Topamax	topiramate
Toprol	metoprolol
Travatan	travoprost
Tricor	fenofibrate
Valtrex	valacyclovir
Viagra	sildenafil
Vicodin	hydrocodone/acetaminophen
Vytorin	ezetimibe/simvastatin
Wellbutrin	bupropion

Brand Name	Generic Name
Xalatan	latanoprost
Zestril	lisinopril
Zetia	ezetimibe
Zithromax	azithromycin
Zocor	simvastatin
Zoloft	sertraline
Zyprexa	olanzapine
Zyrtec	cetirizine

Body Systems

Nervous System

The nervous system is actually comprised of two systems: the **central nervous system** (CNS) and the **peripheral nervous system** (PNS). The two primary organs in the CNS are the **spinal cord** and the **brain**. The rest of the nerves in the body make up the PNS. The purpose of the nervous system is to send impulses to the brain from the nerves and from the brain to the nerves. The brain itself is made up of three separate sections: the **forebrain**, which contains most of the information that makes an individual unique; the **midbrain**, which acts as a controller for the signals traveling to and from the brain along the spinal cord; and the **hindbrain**, which is primarily responsible for coordinating movement. Most of the activity in the nervous system is conducted by cells called **neurons**, which are highly specialized based on their specific function, that transmit signals through an extremely complex chemical process.

Immune System

The immune system is responsible for fighting disease within the body and keeping it healthy and free from infection. The primary components of the immune system include the thymus, spleen, lymphatic system, white blood cells, and bone marrow. The immune system works together in three distinct ways:

- It works to prevent infections from ever entering the body.
- If a foreign body does enter the body, the immune system works to identify it and then eliminate it.
- If bacteria or a virus is able to get into the body and reproduce, the immune system will fight the infection and eliminate it from the body.

In some cases, the immune system can malfunction and identify the body's own system as foreign contaminants, triggering an **immune response**. These conditions are autoimmune disorders and include diseases such as lupus, rheumatoid arthritis, and multiple sclerosis.

Digestive System

The digestive system provides the rest of the body with energy from food and eliminates the waste products. The primary organs of the digestive system include the mouth, esophagus, stomach, liver, gall bladder, pancreas, small intestine, large intestine, and rectum. As food is eaten, it begins to be broken down while still in the **mouth** by chewing and enzymes in saliva. The food passes through the **esophagus** and into the **stomach**, where it is further broken down by gastric acid. It then enters the **small intestine** where bile, produced by the liver and stored in the gall bladder, works together with digestive enzymes, produced by the pancreas and the intestines themselves, to continue breaking down the food. Some nutrients are also absorbed while in the small intestine.

While in the **large intestine**, water and electrolytes are removed from the food. The remaining waste remains in the **rectum** until it is expelled through the **anus**.

Circulatory System

The circulatory system is primarily composed of the veins, arteries, blood cells, and heart. Oxygenated blood starts in the heart and leaves through the **left ventricle** into the **aorta** (the largest artery). The blood then travels throughout the body utilizing the complex system of **arteries**. Once the oxygen is depleted, the blood returns to the heart through the **veins**, passing through the lungs where carbon dioxide is removed. While in the lungs, the blood receives fresh oxygen before returning to the heart. The heart is a complex organ made up of cardiac muscle, a type of striated involuntary muscle.

Reproductive System

The **male reproductive system** is made up primarily of the penis, scrotum, and testes. The **testes** (or testicles) produce testosterone and sperm. The **scrotum** functions to protect the testicles and maintain proper temperature for sperm development. When a male ejaculates, **semen** (a protective fluid that contains the sperm) is released from the testes and travels through the vas deferens to the urethra, which runs through the center of the prostate gland and out through the **penis**. The **female reproductive system** is comprised of the ovaries, fallopian tubes, uterus, cervix, and vagina. Approximately, once a month, one of the **ovaries** releases and egg that travels through the fallopian tube to the uterus. If the egg is not fertilized, the lining that has built up in preparation for a fertilized egg will be shed through **menstruation**. If sperm fertilizes the egg, it will implant in the **uterus**. Over the next 40 weeks, it will develop into a baby. During a process referred to as labor the baby is born, passing through the **cervix** and **vagina**.

Endocrine System

The endocrine system produces the **hormones** that regulate almost every other organ and system in the body. The endocrine system regulates mood, development, metabolism, growth, tissue function, and more. The endocrine system is comprised of the hypothalamus, pituitary gland, pineal gland, thyroid and parathyroid glands, and adrenal gland. Auxiliary organs that also provide hormones and serve as part of the endocrine system include the heart, kidneys, stomach, pancreas, intestines, testes in males, and ovaries in females. Hormones are released by the glands and travel throughout the body to the cells that have receptors that can accept the hormone and exchange chemical information.

Lymphatic System

The lymphatic system works in tandem with the circulatory system and the immune system to keep the body healthy and fight infection. The lymphatic system is comprised of the tonsils, adenoids, thymus, spleen, lymph nodes, and lymph, a clear fluid that is made up of white blood cells and a protective fluid called chyle. **Lymph** travels through a complex circulatory system made up of the lymph nodes, lymph ducts, and lymph vessels. The **lymph nodes** filter lymph as it passes through. If bacteria or other infectious agents are detected, the nodes swell and produce additional white blood cells to help the immune system fight the infection.

Muscular System

The muscular system is composed of three separate types of muscles: the skeletal muscles, the cardiac muscle, and the smooth (or visceral) muscles. The muscle fibers expand and contract, allowing for movement throughout the body. The human body has approximately 650 different muscles, each of which serves a distinct function.

- **Skeletal muscles** are striated, with bands of light and dark layers. They are attached to the skeleton by tendons and are the muscles that are consciously controlled and exercised.
- **Cardiac muscle** is also striated, but the action of this muscle is not consciously controlled. The heart muscle works to keep blood flowing through the circulatory system. When strenuous exercise occurs, the heart can increase its output by up to five times to keep oxygenated blood flowing to the muscles.
- The **smooth or visceral muscles** are found throughout the systems of the body and work to keep the blood vessels and other organs working properly. These muscles are not under conscious control.

Skeletal System

The skeletal system provides a stable framework and support for your body. Certain **bone structures**, such as the skull, ribs, and pelvis also provide protection to the body's most vital organs, such as the brain, heart, and lungs. Additionally, the **tendons** connect the muscles to the bones, which allows for movement. The major bone structures that make up the skeletal system are the skull, spine, ribs, humerus, radius and ulna, pelvis, femur, fibula, and tibia. The bones are made up of several layers. A dense outer layer covers a flexible and spongy layer. The **bone marrow**, which runs through the center of many bones in the skeleton, creates new cells for the blood and provides crucial immune function.

Urinary System

The urinary system is primarily composed of the kidneys, ureters, bladder, and urethra. The **kidneys'** main function is to filter waste from the blood and produce urine. The urine travels from the kidneys through the **ureters** to be held in the bladder until it can be expelled through the **urethra**. The **bladder** contains nerves that signal the brain when the bladder is full and urination to empty the bladder is necessary. **Sphincter muscles** control the opening of the bladder and allow the body to hold onto the urine in the bladder without it leaking out.

Type 2 Diabetes

The risk factors for **Type 2 diabetes** are:

- Excess weight
- Hypertension
- Prediabetes or impaired glucose tolerance
- A sedentary lifestyle
- Insulin resistance
- Genetics
- Ethnic background (diabetes is more common in those of Hispanic, African, Native American, and Asian descent)
- Increased age
- History of gestational diabetes
- Polycystic ovary syndrome

Patients who have these risk factors may be able to **reverse** the likelihood of developing Type 2 diabetes by losing weight and making lifestyle changes. Even once diagnosed, lifestyle change and weight loss can prevent diabetes from progressing and may allow the patient to manage diabetes without the need for medication. Counseling can help patients learn healthier habits.

Rosiglitazone, Metformin, Glargine, and Detemir

Rosiglitazone, metformin, glargine, and detemir are all used to treat diabetes. **Diabetes** is a chronic condition in which the body is unable to stabilize the levels of sugar in the blood because either the body is not making enough **insulin** or the body has built up a resistance to insulin. Diabetes comes in two different forms: Type 1 diabetes and Type 2 diabetes. **Type 1 diabetes** most commonly has an onset in early childhood. **Type 2 diabetes** develops later in life and is often connected to poor diet and exercise habits, although there is also believed to be a genetic component. While diabetes usually does not cause symptoms in day-to-day life, symptoms occur when the blood sugar gets too high or too low. Some of these symptoms include feelings of thirst or hunger, fatigue, blurred eyesight, a tingling sensation in the feet, and increased urination.

Type 2 Diabetes Drug and Non-Drug Therapy

Type 2 diabetes is most effectively treated with a combination of drug and non-drug therapy. **Drug therapy** helps the pancreas produce more insulin or helps the body more effectively use the insulin produced by the pancreas, but this is only part of the treatment. **Non-drug therapy** including dietary and lifestyle counseling is also necessary. Patients with Type 2 diabetes should work to reduce their intake of excess calories, especially those in the form of saturated fat and simple carbohydrates. They should also work on increasing their level of activity. These changes can help fight diabetes and prevent complications due to high blood sugar. They may even reduce the necessity for medication.

Checking Blood Sugar

Patients with diabetes need to test their **blood sugar** on a regular basis to make sure that it is in control. Fluctuating blood sugar levels indicate that a patient's diabetes may not be properly controlled. Most **blood glucose monitors** work in a similar fashion. The patient pricks a finger with a lancet and then applies a drop of blood to a testing strip. The testing strip is then inserted into the meter, which provides a reading of the blood sugar level. Most modern machines require a very small amount of blood for an accurate reading and can provide the result in just seconds. More advanced meters will also store readings for a period of time so that the patient's doctor can see whether the patient's blood sugar levels have been under control.

Review Video: Blood Glucose Pattern Management
Visit mometrix.com/academy and enter code: 626814

Heart Disease

The risk factors for heart disease include:

- Being male, although a woman's risk goes up following menopause
- Increased age
- Genetics
- Ethnicity (heart disease is more common in those of African, Native American, or Hispanic descent)
- Smoking
- High LDL cholesterol
- High blood pressure
- A sedentary lifestyle
- Poorly controlled diabetes
- High levels of stress and anger
- High C-reactive protein

While patients cannot change their ethnicity, age, or family history, many changes can be made to help reduce the risk of heart disease. Quitting **smoking**, eating a diet low in **saturated fat and cholesterol**, and learning better ways to cope with **stress** will all help reduce the risk of developing heart disease.

Review Video: Congestive Heart Failure
Visit mometrix.com/academy and enter code: 924118

High Cholesterol

The risk factors for high cholesterol are:

- Gender (a woman's LDL level increases following menopause)
- A diet high in saturated fat and cholesterol
- Increased age
- Excess weight
- A sedentary lifestyle

While some people develop high cholesterol through genetic factors, many others develop high cholesterol through lifestyle choices. By making significant **lifestyle choices**, including increasing exercise and eating foods low in saturated fat and cholesterol, high cholesterol can be reversed. When LDLs are too high and HDLs are too low, improving the **ratio of LDLs to HDLs** can also be helpful. Eating fatty fish, which are high in omega-3s, and consuming olive oil, a monounsaturated fat, and getting plenty of exercise will help improve your LDL to HDL ratio.

Simvastatin, Pravastatin, Atorvastatin, and Rosuvastatin

Simvastatin, pravastatin, atorvastatin, and rosuvastatin are all used to treat high cholesterol. **High cholesterol** rarely produces any symptoms, but the condition causes fatty deposits to build up in the blood vessels. Over time, these deposits impede the flow of blood through the vessels. When the blood flow to the heart is decreased, a **heart attack** can be the result. When the blood flow to the brain is decreased, a **stroke** may occur. While high cholesterol has a genetic component, eating right and exercise can go a long way toward preventing it. The total cholesterol number is made up of two components: **high-density lipoproteins** (HDL), or good cholesterol, and **low-density lipoproteins** (LDL), or bad cholesterol. While it is helpful to maintain a lower total cholesterol level, it is more important to keep the ratio of HDL to LDL high.

Statin Medications

The class of medications known as statins are used to treat **high cholesterol**. Drinking grapefruit juice or eating large quantities of grapefruit should be avoided while taking this medication. **Grapefruit juice** keeps your body from correctly breaking down the medications, which can cause the statin to build up in your body. This increases the risk of serious side effects such as muscle damage or liver damage. The patient should receive counseling from the pharmacist about avoiding grapefruit juice while taking statin medications. While an increase in dosage may seem like a beneficial thing, too much of the medication is difficult for the liver to process. A symptom of muscle damage is sudden pain in the muscles and should be assessed immediately by a medical provider.

Rhabdomyolysis

Rhabdomyolysis is a serious and potentially deadly side effect that has been linked to statin medications. In this condition, skeletal muscle tissue is quickly broken down and destroyed. All patients receiving statin medications should be counseled on the importance of having recommended blood tests as well as to report any symptoms of muscle pain or fatigue to their doctors, promptly. Undetected and untreated rhabdomyolysis is likely to be **fatal**. While statins are most famously linked, other medications with a connection to rhabdomyolysis include medications for Parkinson's disease, anesthetics, colchicine, and some HIV medications.

High Blood Pressure

High blood pressure has the following risk factors:

- Increased age
- Ethnicity (African Americans are more likely to develop high blood pressure)
- Genetics
- Excess weight
- A sedentary lifestyle
- Tobacco use
- Excess dietary sodium
- Not enough dietary potassium
- Excess use of alcohol
- High stress levels
- Other chronic conditions including diabetes, high cholesterol, kidney disease, and sleep apnea

Because high blood pressure is a risk factor for serious conditions including heart disease and stroke, it is important to keep blood pressure under control. Quitting smoking, losing weight, eating a healthy diet, and exercising regularly are all steps that patients can take to **lower blood pressure**.

Metoprolol, Amlodipine, Valsartan, and Lisinopril

Metoprolol, amlodipine, valsartan, and lisinopril are all intended to treat high blood pressure. **High blood pressure** is a common but serious condition that puts strain on many parts of the body. It is usually not symptomatic, although some people do feel dizzy or have headaches. Untreated high blood pressure leads to coronary artery disease, heart failure, kidney failure, or strokes. Blood pressure is made up of two numbers, **systolic** (the top number) and **diastolic** (the bottom number). A normal blood pressure for adults is a systolic pressure of less than 120 mmHg (millimeters of mercury) and a diastolic of less than 80 mmHg. High blood pressure comes in three stages:

- **Prehypertension** (systolic of 120 – 139 and diastolic of 80 – 89)
- **Stage 1** (systolic of 150 – 159 and diastolic of 90 – 99)
- **Stage 2** (systolic of 160 or higher and diastolic of 100 or higher)

Antihypertensive Medications

The typical dosage range, dosage forms, and routes of administration for the following antihypertensive medications are:

1. **Hydrochlorothiazide** – The recommended dosage for HCTZ is 25 mg to 100 mg per day. It may be taken as a single dose or divided throughout the day. HCTZ is available as an oral capsule, oral tablets, and oral solution.
2. **Atenolol** – Depending on the condition, atenolol is typically dosed at 50 mg to 100 mg daily, up to a maximum of 200 mg daily. Atenolol is available as oral tablets and IV injection.

Amlodipine – Amlodipine may be dosed from 2.5 mg daily to a maximum of 10 mg daily. It is available as an oral tablet.

Benazepril – Typical daily doses of benazepril range from 5 mg to a maximum of 80 mg. Benazepril is available as an oral tablet.

Losartan – Losartan is typically dosed at 25 to 100 mg per day, it may be taken in a single daily dose or divided into two doses. It is available as an oral tablet.

ACE Inhibitors

Angiotensin converting enzyme inhibitors, known as **ACE inhibitors**, treat hypertension and congestive heart failure. As indicated in the name, the medication inhibits the release of angiotensin converting enzyme. This allows for a decrease in blood volume and tension within the vessels, **lowering blood pressure.**

Common ACE inhibitors include:

- Lisinopril
- Enalapril
- Captopril
- Ramipril

Common ACE inhibitor **side effects** include:

- Cough
- Low blood pressure
- Dizziness
- Fatigue
- Headache
- Hyperkalemia

A persistent dry cough is the most common side effect associated with ACE inhibitors. While the cough is not harmful, it can be annoying, and some people may require a different medication to control their hypertension.

Calcium Channel Blockers

Calcium channel blockers work by preventing **calcium** from moving through **calcium channels.** This prevents contraction of vascular smooth muscle, which in turn causes dilation of the blood vessels. This lowers blood pressure and causes the heart to work less. These medications are used to treat hypertension, alter heart rate, and prevent angina.

Common calcium channel blockers include:

- Amlodipine
- Felodipine
- Nifedipine
- Verapamil
- Diltiazem

Side effects associated with calcium channel blockers include:

- Dizziness
- Flushing

- Headache
- Edema
- Tachycardia
- Bradycardia
- Constipation

When used with other medications to treat hypertension, CCB toxicity is a possibility. Some combinations, such as verapamil with beta-blockers, can cause severe bradycardia.

Vasodilators

Vasodilators work by causing dilation of the blood vessels so that blood can flow easily. This decreases the work required by the heart to pump blood throughout the body. Vasodilators treat hypertension, angina, and heart failure. **Nitroglycerin** is the most commonly used vasodilator, and it comes in a variety of forms, including sublingual tablets and sprays, extended release capsules, and transdermal patches and creams. Other vasodilators that may be used include minoxidil and alprostadil, although these medications are also marketed in ways that trade on their side effects (for example, minoxidil for hair regrowth).

Common **side effects** associated with vasodilators include:

- Lightheadedness
- Dizziness
- Low blood pressure
- Flushing

Vasodilators should not be used in combination with certain medications, especially those used to treat erectile dysfunction. This could cause a fatal drop in blood pressure.

Nitroglycerin

Nitroglycerin is a vasodilator that is typically used to relieve episodes of **angina**, or chest pain. Extended release nitroglycerin capsules are taken on a daily basis to prevent recurring angina, while sublingual tablets or sprays are used for occasional occurrences. The medications sildenafil, tadalafil, and vardenafil (typically used for erectile dysfunction) should not be taken concurrently with nitroglycerin. These medications intensify the effect of the nitroglycerin and can cause irreversible **hypotension**, which could be fatal. Should this combination occur accidentally, seek emergency medical care immediately. Symptoms of hypotension include dizziness, fainting, and cold, clammy skin.

Alpha-Agonist Hypotensive Agents

Alpha-agonist hypotensive agents, also called **alpha-blockers**, keep smaller blood vessels open through the relaxing of certain muscles. **Norepinephrine**, a hormone that tightens muscles in the walls of small blood vessels, is blocked, which allows the vessels to remain open and relaxed, decreasing blood pressure. These medications are used to treat **high blood pressure** and **benign prostatic hyperplasia**.

Some examples of alpha agonist hypotensive agents include:

- Doxazosin
- Prazosin

- Tamsulosin
- Alfuzosin

Some common **side effects** associated with alpha-blockers include:

- Low blood pressure
- Dizziness
- Headache
- Pounding heartbeat
- Weakness
- Nausea
- Weight gain
- Decreases in LDL cholesterol

Diuretics

Diuretics are typically used to treat high blood pressure and are associated with a number of common side effects, including:

- **Frequent urination** — Diuretics rid the body of excess water through urination. For this reason, the medication is typically dosed in the morning to avoid disrupting sleep.
- **Abnormalities in electrolytes such as potassium or sodium** — It is important for patients to get regular blood tests as required by their doctor to test for these abnormalities.
- **Fatigue or weakness** —This effect should lessen as the patient becomes used to the medication.
- **Dizziness and lightheadedness** — Postural hypotension (a sudden drop in blood pressure when getting up quickly) is a common side effect when taking diuretics.
- **Dehydration** — If the dose is too high the patient may experience symptoms of dehydration.

Review Video: Diuretics
Visit mometrix.com/academy and enter code: 373276

Loop Diuretics

Loop diuretics specifically target the **loop of Henle**, found in the kidney. The medications inhibit the absorption of sodium and chloride. This prevents concentration of the urine, increasing urine output. The result is a drop in blood volume, **lowering blood pressure** and **reducing edema**.

Loop diuretics include:

- Furosemide
- Torsemide
- Bumetanide

Common **side effects** of loop diuretics are:

- Low levels of other electrolytes such as potassium and magnesium (potassium and magnesium replacements are often prescribed in conjunction with loop diuretics)
- Dehydration
- Dizziness

- Syncope
- Postural hypotension
- Hyperuricemia

Tinnitus and vertigo that occur while taking loop diuretics may be a sign of a serious but rare side effect, ototoxicity, which may result in deafness.

Warfarin

Warfarin is a powerful **blood-thinning agent**. When a patient is taking warfarin, caution is necessary when taking other medications to prevent additional thinning effects, which can have dangerous results. Many pain relievers cause thinning of the blood or can increase the action of the warfarin. Some of these medications include:

- Aspirin
- Acetaminophen
- Ibuprofen
- Naproxen
- Celecoxib
- Diclofenac
- Indomethacin
- Piroxicam

Before taking any medication or making dietary changes, patients who take warfarin will need to speak with a doctor or pharmacist to make sure that the changes are safe. Symptoms that may indicate that blood has become too thin include bleeding that lasts for longer than expected and extensive bruising from relatively small injuries.

Review Video: Warfarin: Most Popular Anticoagulant?
Visit mometrix.com/academy and enter code: 844117

Tachycardia, Bradycardia, and Arrhythmia

Tachycardia means rapid heartbeat and usually indicates a heartbeat that exceeds the normal resting rate. This number can vary greatly depending on the age and fitness level of the individual. Depending on the rate and quality of the rhythm, tachycardia can be dangerous or may be a symptom of a serious health condition. **Bradycardia** means slow heartbeat. In adults, bradycardia is generally considered a heart rate lower than 60 beats per minute (however, this can vary depending on the patient's fitness level and usual resting heart rate). The patient usually remains asymptomatic until the heart rate drops below 50 beats per minute. A low heart rate may indicate or lead to cardiac arrest. **Arrhythmia**, also known as cardiac dysrhythmia, is any unusual heartbeat, including tachycardia, bradycardia, and irregular heartbeats. While some arrhythmias are harmless, others can indicate a serious condition requiring emergency medical treatment.

Depression

Depression is a serious condition and when left untreated could potentially result in the patient's death from **suicide**. Treating depression requires a two-pronged approach. Medication is helpful because it regulates the levels of serotonin, norepinephrine, and dopamine in the brain, but by combining medication with therapy and counseling, the patient is much better equipped to cope with day-to-day life. **Medication** works to correct the chemical imbalances in the brain that cause depression. **Talk therapy** helps the patient to erase negative and defeating thoughts and replace them with positive self-talk and behaviors.

Escitalopram, Venlafaxine, Bupropion, and Sertraline

Escitalopram, venlafaxine, bupropion and sertraline are all intended to treat **depression**, a mood disorder identified by intense feelings of sadness, anger, loss, and frustration. The exact mechanism of depression is unknown, although most researchers believe it to be a combination of **genetic predisposition** and **situational factors**. Depression can happen to anyone regardless of age, race, gender, or social class.

Some of the common symptoms of depression include:

- Difficulty concentrating
- Loss of interest in previously enjoyable activities
- Fatigue
- A sense of worthlessness or hopelessness
- Thoughts of suicide
- Difficulty sleeping

Treatment for depression usually includes a combination of **antidepressants** and **therapy** with a counselor or psychiatrist.

Antidepressants

The typical dosage range, dosage forms, and routes of administration for the following antidepressants are:

1. **Amitriptyline** – Amitriptyline may be started at a dose as low as 10 mg and may be increased to 300 mg per day. It may be taken as a single dose or divided into two to three doses per day. Amitriptyline comes as oral tablets and intramuscular injection.
2. **Bupropion** – The typical adult dose for bupropion is 150 mg to 300 mg per day in divided doses or as a single extended release tablet. The maximum daily dose is 450 mg per day. Bupropion is available as standard and extended release oral tablets.
3. **Citalopram** – Citalopram is dosed at 20 mg to 40 mg per day. Doses above 40 mg daily are not recommended. Citalopram is available as oral tablets or oral solution.
4. **Mirtazapine** – Mirtazapine is typically dosed at 15 mg to 45 mg per day. Mirtazapine is available as oral tablets and disintegrating oral tablets.

MAOI

MAOI stands for **monoamine oxidase inhibitor**. This class of medications is used to treat depression. While these were the first type of **antidepressants** developed, the side effect profile and potential for dangerous interactions is so high that today these medications are only used to treat depression that is resistant to other forms of treatment. Some examples of MAOIs include phenelzine (brand name Nardil), selegiline (brand name Emsam), and tranylcypromine (brand name Parnate). MAOIs can cause a number of side effects including serotonin syndrome, a condition in which the patient's serotonin levels become dangerously high. Symptoms of serotonin syndrome mimic those of a heart attack. Numerous medications and foods can cause severe side effects when taken with MAOIs. Foods containing tyramine, such as wine, cheese, certain meats, and pickled foods, can cause spikes in blood pressure when taken concurrently with MAOIs.

Antipsychotics

The class of atypical antipsychotic medications includes:

- Aripiprazole
- Clozapine
- Olanzapine
- Quetiapine
- Risperidone
- Ziprasidone

These medications are typically used to treat mental illnesses such as **schizophrenia** and **bipolar disorder**. Other uses include treatment of anxiety disorders and obsessive-compulsive disorder. Side effects within this class of medications are variable. One common side effect, and the one that is usually the most concerning, is the risk of developing tardive dyskinesia, a disorder in which the patient displays repetitive, involuntary movements such as twirling of the feet, lip smacking, or eye blinking.

Other possible **side effects** include:

- Dystonia
- Reduction in sexual interest
- Abnormal menstrual cycles
- Enlargement of the breasts
- Increased risk of diabetes
- Weight gain

Esomeprazole, Omeprazole, Lansoprazole, and Pantoprazole

Esomeprazole, omeprazole, lansoprazole, and pantoprazole are all used to treat **gastroesophageal reflux disease**, or **GERD**. In this condition, the lower esophageal sphincter is weak and does not close properly, allowing the contents of the stomach to back up into the esophagus, causing irritation. Some of the common symptoms of GERD include a painful, burning sensation known as heartburn, coughing, nausea, difficulty swallowing, and a hoarse voice. GERD can be caused or exacerbated by a number of factors. Some of these include obesity, pregnancy, overconsumption of foods, highly acidic foods, a hiatal hernia, and smoking. In addition to taking medications, people who suffer from GERD can help keep their condition under control by avoiding triggering foods, losing weight (if obesity is a factor), eating less food at a meal, and avoiding lying down soon after a meal.

Nebulizer

A nebulizer is a device used to aerosolize liquid medications so that a patient can easily **inhale** them. It is usually used to treat patients with asthma or pneumonia. Some medications for inhalers come in premixed concentrations (such as 0.083% albuterol), while other concentrations may require mixing by the patient. The nebulizer consists of the main machine, the filter, tubing, a holding chamber, and the mouthpiece or mask. Each piece will require regular cleaning for the machine to work correctly. Filters especially need to be cleaned or replaced on a regular basis.

Montelukast, Albuterol, Fluticasone, and Budesonide

Montelukast, albuterol, fluticasone, and budesonide are all used to treat **asthma**. Asthma causes swelling in the passages of the lungs, making breathing difficult and leading to such symptoms as wheezing, coughing, chest tightness, and shortness of breath. Asthma is a serious condition and requires prompt treatment. Untreated asthma could lead to death. Asthma can be triggered by a number of factors, including environmental allergies, some medications, stress, smoke, and respiratory infections. Treatment of asthma usually includes a **long-acting control medication** (inhaled corticosteroids like fluticasone or a leukotriene inhibitor like montelukast) and a **fast-acting medication** like albuterol or ipratropium to stop an asthma attack in progress. Other factors in treating asthma include knowing and avoiding triggers, having an asthma plan that directs when to self-treat and when to seek emergency assistance, and tracking breathing using a peak flow meter.

HIV

HIV is the virus that causes **AIDS**, a serious disease in which the body's immune system is destroyed. Although HIV treatment has improved considerably, there is still no known cure for the disease. HIV infection is passed from person to person via contact with bodily fluids.

The most common forms of transmission include:

- Unprotected sexual contact with an infected person
- Sharing needles with an infected person

Children born to infected mothers have the possibility of acquiring the disease. In the healthcare field, contact with **blood** or other **bodily fluids** from an infected person poses a risk of transmission. Medical staff can protect themselves by wearing personal protective equipment such as gloves and masks, following proper infection control procedures, and using caution around needles that have been used to give injections to patients.

Hepatitis B

Hepatitis B is a viral infection that attacks the **liver**, causing inflammation. It can eventually lead to liver failure and death. Hepatitis B is transmitted through contact with bodily fluids, including:

- Unprotected sexual contact
- Tattoos performed with shared instruments
- Sharing needles and other paraphernalia used to inject drugs
- Sharing of personal items such as razors and toothbrushes
- Childbirth

If you are exposed to blood or other bodily fluids while working, notify your infection control team immediately. Because people working in healthcare are considered high risk, you should be **vaccinated** against hepatitis B to prevent contracting the disease.

Antibiotics

The typical dosage range, dosage forms, and routes of administration for the following antibiotics are:

1. **Amoxicillin** — Amoxicillin is typically dosed 250 mg to 500 mg every 8 hours, or 500 to 875 mg every 12 hours. Amoxicillin comes as a chewable tablet, a capsule, and a powder for suspension.
2. **Penicillin VK** — Typical dosing of penicillin VK is 125 mg to 500 mg every 6 to 8 hours. Penicillin VK is available as oral tablets and powder for suspension.
3. **Cephalexin** — Cephalexin doses are typically 250 mg every 6 hours or 500 mg every 12 hours. Cephalexin is available as oral capsules and powder for suspension.

4. **Cefuroxime** — Cefuroxime doses are typically 250 mg to 500 mg every 12 hours. It is available as tablets and as powder for oral suspension.
5. **Azithromycin** — Azithromycin may be taken as a single dose of 1000 mg, three daily doses of 500 mg, or one daily dose of 500 mg followed by four daily doses of 250 mg. It is available as oral tablets or powder for oral suspension.

Amoxicillin, Penicillin, Clarithromycin, Tetracycline, and Cephalexin

These medications are all **antibiotics**. They are used to treat infections caused by bacteria. Antibiotics work to rid the body of infection in one of two ways. Some, such as penicillin, kill the bacteria. Others stop bacteria from multiplying. Antibiotics are ineffective against **viral infections**. The doctor may perform a culture to determine which strain of bacteria is causing the infection, as some bacteria are more susceptible to certain classes of antibiotics. Overuse of antibiotics has become a serious issue in the United States, and there have been many reports of "**superbugs**" — bacteria that have become resistant to all but the most powerful of antibiotics.

Controlled Substances

The typical dosage range, dosage forms, and routes of administration for the following controlled substances are:

1. **Hydrocodone/acetaminophen** — The hydrocodone portion is available in strengths of 2.5 mg to 10 mg and the acetaminophen portion ranges from 325 mg to 650 mg. Doses are typically one or two tablets at various times throughout the day, depending on the severity of the pain. The medication should not exceed a total daily dose of 4000 mg of acetaminophen. This medication comes in oral tablets of varying doses as well as oral solution.
2. **Lorazepam** — Lorazepam is typically taken as needed, up to 6 mg per day in divided doses. Lorazepam is available as an oral tablet and injectable solution
3. **Methylphenidate** — Methylphenidate may be dosed at up to 72 mg per day (available as the brand name Concerta). Immediate release tablets may be taken once or twice daily and extended release formulations are taken once daily. Methylphenidate is available as oral tablets and oral extended release tablets.

Oral Contraceptives

Oral contraceptives are associated with a number of side effects, some of which can be severe. **Birth control pills** increase the risk of potentially deadly blood clots, particularly in women over age 35 or who smoke (women who are 35 years of age or older and smoke should not take oral contraceptives). Common and less severe **side effects** include:

- Nausea
- Weight gain
- Spotting between periods
- Changes in mood
- Lighter periods
- Aching or swollen breasts

Serious side effects that require immediate emergency care include:

- Chest pain
- Blurred vision

- Stomach pain
- Severe headaches

Yasmin, Ortho Tri-Cyclen, Trinessa, Sprintec, and Ovcon

Yasmin, Ortho Tri-Cyclen, TriNessa, Sprintec, and Ovcon are all **oral contraceptives**, and are often referred to as birth control pills or simply "**the pill**." They are taken on a daily basis by women to avoid pregnancy. Oral contraceptives work in a number of ways to prevent pregnancy. Oral contraceptives contain **estrogen** and/or **progestin** (progestin only oral contraceptives include Micronor and Ovrette and are often known as the "minipill"). By supplying a steady stream of these hormones, the hormones that cause eggs to mature and to be released from the ovary are suppressed. Additionally, the hormones prevent the **endometrium** from thickening enough to support a fertilized egg. **Progestins** create a mucus barrier, which prevents the sperm from reaching an egg to fertilize it. It is also believed that progestins cause changes to the **fallopian tubes** that make it difficult for an egg to pass through them.

Birth Control

Antibiotics have been known to reduce or disrupt the action of **hormonal birth control**. This means that a woman taking **oral contraceptives** (or other hormonal methods such as NuvaRing) may become pregnant if also taking an **antibiotic**. Pharmacists should always counsel women taking antibiotics about this concern, as the patient might be receiving birth control through another pharmacy or source. A barrier method, such as condoms, must be used during the course of antibiotics and for at least two weeks afterward to prevent an unwanted pregnancy. Other drugs that may affect birth control include anti-fungal medications, some anti-seizure medications, certain HIV medications, and some herbal preparations such as St. John's Wort.

Antihistamines

Although many antihistamines are available over the counter, they still have a number of **side effects**. These side effects include:

- Drowsiness (this side effect is very common, and many antihistamines, such as diphenhydramine, are marketed under different trade names as sleep aids. Antihistamines should not be taken when it is necessary to be alert and especially should not be taken before driving.)
- Headaches
- Increased blood pressure
- Stomach upset

Dry mouth and decreased urination (the anticholinergic effect of antihistamines that makes them useful for drying up a stuffy nose can also cause drying in other areas of the body).

Potential Side Effects of Chemotherapy

Although chemotherapy is often effective for treating cancer, it is also known for having considerable **side effects**. Medication is frequently prescribed along with chemotherapy to help counter these side effects. Some common side effects include:

- Constipation or diarrhea (laxatives or anti-diarrhea medications such as loperamide are often prescribed concurrently with chemotherapy)
- Fatigue
- Hair Loss
- Weakened immune system leading to infection

- Anemia (IV drugs to support red blood cell development such as darbepoetin alfa may be prescribed)
- Loss of appetite (medications such as dronabinol can help stimulate appetite)
- Nausea and vomiting (anti-emetics and anti-nausea medications like promethazine or ondansetron are often prescribed)
- Neuropathy
- Pain
- Fluid retention

Total Parenteral Nutrition

Total parenteral nutrition may be used under a variety of different circumstances. Some of the most common include:

- Malnourishment due to any cause
- Liver or kidney failure
- Short bowel syndrome
- Severe burns
- Enterocutaneous fistulas
- Sepsis
- Chemotherapy and radiation
- Neonates
- Any condition requiring full bowel rest, which may include pancreatitis, ulcerative colitis, or Crohn's disease

Essentially, any situation in which the patient is unable to take food orally or digest food through the stomach and intestines may indicate the use of total parenteral nutrition. The goal is to keep the patient nourished to prevent **wasting** or **malnutrition**.

Possible Complications with Total Parenteral Nutrition

Although total parenteral nutrition is a good way to keep patients nourished when they are unable to eat on their own, some **complications** are possible, and providers should watch their patients carefully to make sure that they do not develop one of these conditions:

- Acidosis
- Calcification of the vena cava
- Electrolyte imbalances
- Glycemic imbalances, such as hyperglycemia or hypoglycemia
- Hematoma
- Liver dysfunction
- Pneumothorax
- Infection at the catheter site
- Triglyceride imbalances

Proper **monitoring of blood work** will help prevent or quickly detect most of these conditions, which can then be remedied through medication or adjusting the TPN formula.

Sympathomimetic Agents

Sympathomimetic drugs work by mimicking the body's natural sympathetic nervous response system, which produces such transmitters as **epinephrine**, **norepinephrine**, and **dopamine**.

These medications are often given in emergencies to treat cardiac arrest and shock. They are also used to treat dangerously low blood pressure and prevent premature labor. Many stimulants used to treat attention-deficit disorder are also sympathomimetic in nature.

Medications classified as sympathomimetic drugs include:

- Ephedrine
- Methylphenidate
- Pemoline
- Caffeine
- Dobutamine
- Dopamine
- Terbutaline

Side effects associated with these drugs include:

- Hypertension
- Cardiac arrhythmia
- Nervousness
- Headache
- Anxiety
- Dilated pupils
- Vertigo

Benzodiazepines

Benzodiazepines enhance the effect of the neurotransmitter **GABA**, producing a central nervous system **depressant** effect. While these medications eventually replaced the more dangerous barbiturate class of medication, they still are known for causing significant physical dependence and withdrawal symptoms. Benzodiazepines are used as sedatives and hypnotics, as well as in anticonvulsive therapy. Some benzodiazepines are used to assist with the symptoms of alcohol withdrawal. Most barbiturates are classified as CIV controlled substances. Commonly used benzodiazepines include:

- Diazepam
- Lorazepam
- Clonazepam
- Alprazolam
- Midazolam
- Temazepam

Side effects of benzodiazepines include:

- Physical dependence
- Sedation
- Drowsiness
- Dizziness
- Lack of coordination

Methotrexate

Methotrexate is a medication used to treat severe psoriasis, rheumatoid arthritis, and certain types of cancer including breast cancer, lung cancer, lymphoma, and leukemia. Methotrexate is in the class of medications called **antimetabolites**. It works to slow the growth of abnormal cells and impedes the action of the immune system. Methotrexate has a number of **side effects**, some of which are potentially dangerous, including:

- Dizziness
- Drowsiness
- Headache
- Swollen gums
- Increased chance of infection
- Hair loss
- Confusion
- Weakness

Methotrexate is prescribed in **weekly bursts** and should not be taken as a daily medication. Dosing errors associated with methotrexate can be deadly. If a prescription is written for daily methotrexate, bring it to the pharmacist's attention immediately so that the doctor can be contacted. Signage in the pharmacy to remind staff of this dosing requirement can help prevent dangerous mistakes.

Corticosteroids

Corticosteroids are a large group of medications used to treat a number of different conditions involving swelling and inflammation. Corticosteroids, although synthetic, are similar to naturally produced **cortisol**. Corticosteroid medications may be taken orally, used as nasal sprays, ocular and aural drops, topical creams and ointments, inhalants, or injections. They are used to treat a variety of conditions from asthma to skin rashes to arthritis.

Some examples of commonly used corticosteroids include:

- Prednisone
- Hydrocortisone
- Triamcinolone
- Mometasone
- Budesonide
- Fluocinolone
- Betamethasone
- Dexamethasone

Prolonged use of corticosteroids can be dangerous, especially when used topically. It can cause damage to healthy tissue. Other **side effects** associated with corticosteroids include:

- Insulin resistance and diabetes
- Osteoporosis
- Depression
- Hypertension
- Hypothyroidism

Smoking Cessation

Smoking is one of the leading causes of numerous serious conditions, including heart disease and cancer. Quitting smoking is one of the most important things someone can do for his or her health; however, the difficulty in fighting a **nicotine addiction** is also recognized. While ongoing support and behavioral modification therapy are helpful when quitting, many medications including bupropion (marketed as Zyban) and varenicline (Chantix) can make it easier to fight the urge to smoke. Additionally, **nicotine replacement systems** including gum, patches, and lozenges can help patients cope with the cravings while they are quitting. **Support** from friends and family can be the most powerful assistance of all when it comes to quitting smoking.

Acetaminophen Dosage

For people with healthy livers, the maximum daily dose of **acetaminophen** is **4,000 mg per day**. For people with compromised livers due to alcoholism or liver disease, the maximum dose is **2,000 mg per day** or less. Some people with liver disease may not be able to take acetaminophen at all. Acetaminophen is primarily metabolized in the **liver**. When the liver is inundated with too much acetaminophen, the pathways through which it is metabolized become saturated, the liver is unable to keep up, and the acetaminophen is processed through a different pathway. When this occurs, the by-product is toxic. The **toxic compound** builds up in the liver, and damage occurs.

Alcohol and Medications

Alcohol should be avoided while taking most medications. The side effects can vary based on the medication. In some cases, alcohol combined with medications can cause nausea and vomiting, fainting, loss of coordination, or extreme drowsiness. A more serious reaction can lead to heart problems, internal bleeding, and difficulty breathing. Some medications combined with alcohol can create a toxic combination. Alcohol is a strong **CNS depressant**. Combining alcohol with other depressants, such as benzodiazepines or sleeping medications can pose a serious risk and can cause patients to stop breathing. Combining alcohol with acetaminophen can cause serious liver damage. When taking metronidazole, alcohol causes serious illness including nausea and vomiting and liver damage.

Hypertension and Medications

Many over-the-counter medications can cause a rise in **blood pressure**, which can be dangerous in patients with **hypertension**. Some of the medications known to be problematic for patients with hypertension include **NSAIDs** such as ibuprofen and naproxen, decongestants such as pseudoephedrine, weight loss formulas and supplements, and migraine formulations that contain caffeine. Patients with high blood pressure should check with a doctor or pharmacist before taking any medications or herbal supplements. Symptoms of high blood pressure include headache, dizziness, and shortness of breath. Instruct patients to keep track of their blood pressure on a regular basis. Note any sudden change and notify their medical provider immediately.

Converting Teaspoon and Tablespoon Measurements into Milliliters

When dosing medications, a **teaspoon** is equivalent to **5 mL**, and a **tablespoon** is equivalent to **15 mL**. The pharmacist should counsel patients on how to dose liquid medications properly using a specially marked spoon or oral syringe. Patients should be advised to never dose medications using spoons intended for eating, despite the teaspoon and tablespoon name, as sizes vary.

2 tsp. = 10 mL
2 tbsp. = 30 mL
4 tbsp. = 60 mL
1.5 tsp. = 7.5 mL

0.5 tbsp. = 7.5 mL
20 mL = 4 tsp.
2.5 mL = 0.5 tsp.

Converting Milliliters into Ounces

One **liquid ounce** is equivalent to **30 mL**. When measuring liquid medications for dispensing, use a graduated cylinder, and pour slowly to measure the correct amount.

180 mL = 6 ounces
240 mL = 8 ounces
90 mL = 3 ounces
2 ounces = 60 mL
12 ounces = 360 mL
5 ounces = 150 mL

Ratio of Cups to Pints to Quarts to Gallons

Two **cups** are in one **pint**. Two pints are in one **quart**. Four quarts are in one **gallon**. Because one cup contains eight **ounces**:

One pint is 16 ounces.
One quart is 32 ounces.
One gallon is 128 ounces.

Conversion of Grams to Pounds

One **kilogram** (1000 grams) is equivalent to **2.2 pounds**.

1 pound = 454 grams
2 pounds = 908 grams
227 grams = 0.5 pounds
681 grams = 1.5 pounds

Conversion of Grams to Ounces

A **dry ounce** is equivalent to **30 grams**.

15 grams = 0.5 ounce
60 grams = 2 ounces
120 grams = 4 ounces
1.5 ounces = 45 grams
3 ounces = 90 grams

Conversion of Drops to Milliliters

Each **mL** contains **20 drops**.

5 gtt ou bid x 10 days =10 ml (5 drops in each eye twice daily for 10 days)

1 gtt au tid x 30 days = 9 ml (1 drop in each ear three times daily for 30 days)

2 gtt os qd x 15 days = 1.5 mL (2 drops in left eye daily for 15 days)

1 gtt ou q2h x 5 days = 6 mL (1 drop in both eyes every 2 hours for 5 days)

3 gtt sl q4h x 7 days = 6.3 mL (3 drops sublingually every 4 hours for 7 days)

Most medications dispensed in drops come in standard sized bottles (such as 10 mL or 15 mL). The entire bottle is dispensed, even if it is more than the required days' supply. It is still necessary to calculate days' supply, for both insurance purposes and to know how many or which size bottle to dispense.

Conversion of Grains to Milligrams

One **grain** is equivalent to **65 milligrams.**

2 grains = 130 mg
1.5 grains = 97.5 mg
0.5 grains = 32.5 mg
325 mg = 5 grains
650 mg = 10 grains
162.5 mg = 2.5 grains

Celsius and Fahrenheit Temperatures Conversions

The formula for converting **Fahrenheit to Celsius** is:

$$C = (F - 32) \text{ x } \left(\frac{5}{9}\right)$$

The formula for converting **Celsius to Fahrenheit** is:

$$F = C \text{ x } (9/5) + 32$$

Examples

40 °F	=	4.45 °C
67 °F	=	19.46 °C
98.6 °F	=	37 °C
102 °F	=	38.89 °C
10 °C	=	50 °F
50 °C	=	122 °F

Pediatric Dose Rules

Young's rule relies on age to calculate the dose, using the formula

$$\text{adult dose} \times \left(\frac{\text{age}}{\text{age} + 12}\right) = \text{pediatric dose}$$

Drilling's rule also relies on age. The formula used in this rule is

$$\frac{\text{age} \times \text{adult dose}}{12} = \text{pediatric dose}$$

Fried's rule uses the child's age in months, with the formula

$$\frac{\text{age in months} \times \text{adult dose}}{150} = \text{pediatric dose}$$

Clark's rule is based on the child's weight in pounds, using the formula

$$\frac{\text{weight in pounds} \times \text{adultdose}}{150} = \text{pediactric dose}$$

Proportional Calculation

Proportional calculations are used frequently in the pharmacy. They may be used to determine how much medication should be dispensed, to calculate a dose, or in compounding. A proportional calculation is typically set up as:

$$\frac{a}{b} = \frac{c}{d}$$

In a simple scenario, the technician may have received the following prescription: Amoxicillin suspension, 250 mg bid x 10 days. Upon checking the shelf, the only concentration available is 200 mg/5 ml. To calculate the dose, set the equation up:

$$\frac{200\ \text{mg}}{5\ \text{ml}} = \frac{250\ \text{mg}}{x}$$

To solve for x, multiply 5 by 250, then divide by 200. The answer is 6.25 ml. When performing these calculations, be careful to use the **same units of measurement**. If one side is in mg/ml and the other is in mcg/ml, the math will be incorrect. One will need to be converted for the units to be the same.

Proportion Technique

To solve dilution problems using **proportion technique**, the steps are as follows:

- Setting up your proportion equation: $\left(\frac{\text{x}}{\text{total}}\right) = \left(\frac{\text{percentage}}{100}\right)$
- Solve for x for the total number of units of active ingredient in the solution.
- Determine the quantity of diluted solution to be made using proportions:

$$\frac{\text{active ingredient}}{\text{x}} = \frac{\text{desired dilution percentage}}{100}$$

- Solve for x to get the total quantity of diluted solution you can make.
- Determine how much diluent to add by subtracting the original amount of solution you had from the total amount of diluted solution.

Explain how proportion technique is used to determine dilutions of solutions and solve the following problem: How much sterile water would you use to dilute 1 L of 70% alcohol percent solution to 40% solution? How much total 40% solution would you make?

To solve the problem:

$$\frac{x\ \text{mL}}{1000\ \text{mL}} = \frac{70}{100}$$

Solve for x:

$$\frac{1000\ x\ 70}{100} = x$$

The solution contains 700 ml of alcohol.

$$\frac{700}{x} = \frac{40}{100}$$

Solve for x:

$$\frac{700\ x\ 100}{40} = x$$

The total amount of diluted solution that can be made is 1750 ml. To get this solution, add 750 ml of sterile water.

V/V, W/W, and W/V Concentrations

Concentrations may be expressed as a **ratio** of ingredients or as a **percentage**. In concentrations, V/V, W/W, and W/V are used to indicate **ratios of solute**, or drug, to solvent. V/V represents a volume/volume ratio, and the unit used in this measurement is mL. W/W represents a weight/weight ratio, and the unit used in this measurement is grams. W/V is used to indicate a weight/volume ratio, and the measurement used is grams/mL.

1. V/V = 1:200 = 1 mL/200 mL = 0.5%
2. W/W = 3:100 = 3 grams/100 grams = 3%
3. W/V = 15/100 = 15 grams/100 mL = 15%

Alligation Method

The alligation method is often referred to as the "Tic-Tac-Toe" method because the problems are set up on a grid that resembles a tic-tac-toe grid.

Set up the problem by placing the concentration you want in the middle box, the higher concentration you have in stock in the upper left hand corner, and the lower concentration you have in stock in the lower left hand corner. Move from the lower left hand corner to the upper right hand corner. The difference between the number in the lower left hand corner and the number in the middle box goes in the upper right hand corner. Moving from the upper left hand corner to the lower right hand corner, the difference between the number in the upper left hand corner and the number in the middle goes in the lower right hand corner. The number on the right represents the parts of the concentration across from it on the left that are used to create the needed concentration. **Proportion math** will help you determine how much of each to use.

Problem

The pharmacist has instructed you to mix 0.75 L of a 70% alcohol solution with 1.5 L of a 40% alcohol solution. Show the strength of the final solution.

This type of problem is referred to as a $C_1V_1 = C_2V_2$ problem, with C standing for **concentration** and V standing for **volume**. The numbers refer to each solution in the combination. Set up the equation to solve the problem as:

$$C_1V_1 + C_2V_2 = C_FV_F$$

To solve the problem provided, set up the equation as:

$$0.7(750\ mL) + 0.4(1500\ mL) = C_F(2250\ mL)$$

Solve the problem for C_F:

$$525\ mL + 600\ mL = C_F(2250\ mL)$$

$$\frac{1125}{2250} = C_F$$

$$C_F = 0.5$$

Which means the strength of the finished solution will be 50%.

Sample Algebra Problems

Sample 1

If your wholesale price of 50 mg Zoloft is $4 per tablet and a patient brings in a prescription for 30 tablets, how much will the script cost the patient if you include a 50% markup over wholesale and a $3 dispensing fee?

First determine the total wholesale price: $4 x 30 = $120. Now, add in the markup, $120 x 1.50 = $180. Add in your dispensing fee, $180 + $3 = $183 is the total retail price for 30 tablets of 50 mg Zoloft.

Sample 2

If you are working in a pharmacy that sells 30 10 mg Norvasc tablets for $110 and you know that your typical markup is 40% over wholesale and you add on a $6 dispensing fee to every prescription, what is the wholesale price your pharmacy pays for each tablet of Norvasc?

To solve this problem, begin by subtracting the dispensing fee from the total: $110 – $6 = $104. To reverse the markup, divide $104 by 1.40 (the 1 in 1.40 represents the 100% of the markup price) = $74.28. Now divide by the quantity, $74.28/30 = $2.47. Your pharmacy is paying $2.47 for each tablet of 10 mg Norvasc.

Durable vs. Non-Durable Medical Equipment

Durable medical equipment is any device used to treat a medical condition that is not disposable. Examples include wheelchairs, walkers, diabetic blood testing monitors, home oxygen equipment, nebulizers, prosthetics, slings, braces, and orthotics. **Non-durable medical equipment** is a product used to treat a medical condition that is intended to be disposable or is not intended for more than one use. Examples include diabetic testing supplies such as lancets and test strips, insulin syringes and needles, casts, catheters, and ostomy supplies.

Blood Pressure Monitors

A number of different **blood pressure monitors** are available to the public. Standard cuffs that fit over the arm are available as are varieties that fit over the wrist. Some cuffs inflate automatically while some need to be manually inflated. Advanced models of blood pressure monitors not only inflate automatically, but also store your readings, allowing them to be easily viewed and tracked by you and your doctor. Most experts consider **upper arm monitors** to be more accurate than **wrist monitors**. Readings on wrist monitors can vary greatly depending on the position of the arm and wrist, so it is important to read and follow the manufacturer's directions for use. To test a wrist monitor for accuracy, a patient can take it with him or her to a doctor appointment and check his or her blood pressure on both the wrist monitor and the doctor's equipment.

Orthopedic Supplies

Orthopedic supplies include such devices as braces, crutches, splints, insoles, and more. Most of these devices are intended to position **stabilize** the affected body part to allow healing or prevent injury. Knee and ankle braces are two braces commonly used for that purpose. Wrist and thumb braces treat and prevent conditions like carpal tunnel syndrome. A broken limb may require a sling or splint to keep the area immobile to ensure proper healing. Crutches help patients with leg, ankle, or foot injuries keep weight off the affected area.

Ostomy Supplies

Ostomy supplies are used following surgery that requires moving part of the **colon** or **bladder**. Ostomy supplies include adhesive wafers, skin protectants, deodorants, and collection bags that hold waste products that would otherwise be stored in the bladder or colon. Patients with an ostomy will have an opening in their body called a **stoma**. A collection bag with an adhesive ring (sometimes called a wafer) attaches to the skin around the stoma to collect the waste products. Many of these products are carried in pharmacies or can be specifically ordered for patients. It is important to know which type of ostomy surgery a patient has had (**colostomy**, **urostomy**, or **ileostomy**) so that the right supplies can be ordered.

Insulin Pump

Some people with Type 1 diabetes have a hard time keeping blood sugar under control and may require frequent **injections** of insulin. For these patients, an **insulin pump** that provides continuous insulin infusion throughout the day is a better solution than frequent injections that can cause blood sugar highs and lows. An insulin pump includes a few different pieces and supplies, including the pump itself, an insulin reservoir, a subcutaneous cannula, and tubing system. The reservoir, cannula, and tubing system are replaceable and are carried in many pharmacies or can be ordered. Insulin pumps are programmed by the doctor to deliver specific doses of insulin at specific times to keep the patient's blood sugar stable.

Crash Cart

A crash cart, also called a **code cart**, is a cart located in several locations throughout hospitals or other medical centers to be used in case of a cardiac emergency or other emergencies in which the patient requires **resuscitation**. The crash cart contains medical supplies and medications necessary for resuscitation, including:

- Heart rate monitors
- Defibrillators
- Intubating equipment and medications used during intubation: succinylcholine (a paralytic), etomidate, midazolam, or another sedative
- Advanced Cardiac Life Support Drugs such as amiodarone, atropine, dopamine, epinephrine, lidocaine, sodium bicarbonate, and vasopressin
- Other drugs that may be included are adenosine, dextrose, diazepam, naloxone, or nitroglycerin

Code Blue

Code Blue is used in many hospitals and medical centers throughout the country to indicate a medical emergency in which **resuscitation** is immediately necessary. The most common conditions requiring a Code Blue call are **cardiac or respiratory arrest**. Code Blue, along with the exact location of the patient, is announced on the hospital intercom system. This is the signal for those personnel assigned to respond to emergencies to arrive on location as quickly as possible. The pharmacy will usually have staff, often a pharmacist and technician, assigned to respond to a Code Blue. Responsibilities will vary by location, so know your location's policy. Pharmacy staff may be required to bring necessary medication or to call for supplies if they should run low. Technicians will be called upon to restock the crash cart following a Code Blue.

Intubation

Intubation involves the insertion of a tube into the **trachea** via the mouth or nose. In emergencies, it might also be done via tracheotomy or other surgical procedures. Intubation is done for a variety of reasons:

- To maintain an open airway
- To administer some types of medication
- To facilitate lung ventilation
- To prevent asphyxiation

Certain medications are given during intubation, as it is an invasive and uncomfortable procedure. Paralytics such as succinylcholine are used, as well as sedatives such as midazolam or etomidate. Preferably, the person undergoing intubation will be under general anesthesia, although it can be performed while the patient is awake, if necessary.

CPR

Cardiopulmonary resuscitation (or CPR) is used on an emergency basis to assist patients who are not breathing or whose heart has stopped beating. The compressions simulate heartbeats to help keep blood moving throughout the body, preventing brain damage until the heart can restart. By providing **artificial respiration**, air is forced into the lungs. The goal of CPR is not to restart the heart; it is to keep the tissue from dying and extend the person's chances for survival. In adults, a ratio of 30 compressions to two breaths is used. In children, the ratio is 15:2. The acronym CAB can be used to remember the order: **compressions**, **airway**, and **breathing**. Perform compressions at a rate of 100 compressions per minute at a depth of about five cm. All personnel in every healthcare setting should obtain and maintain CPR certification bi-annually.

Heimlich Maneuver

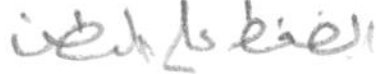

The Heimlich Maneuver is used to help people who are **choking**. The maneuver helps to dislodge the food or object that is caught in the airway. The procedure is performed as follows:

- Stand behind the victim, and wrap your arms around him or her.
- Making a fist, position the thumb side of the fist so that it is pressing into the abdomen, above the navel and below the rib cage.
- Holding the fist with the other hand, perform a quick, upward thrust, driving the fist into the upper abdomen.
- Repeat until the object is expelled.
- Heimlich Maneuver training is often included in CPR training programs.

Standard Hospital Emergency Codes

While no standard system from hospital to hospital yet exists, certain issues may present themselves in hospitals and medical centers. It is important to learn the **codes** used to identify these situations and to know your role in them, should one occur. Some possibilities are:

- **Code Blue** – often used to identify a cardiac or respiratory emergency
- **Bomb threat** – keep the caller on the phone while contacting security
- **Child abduction** – often identified by Amber Alert or Code Pink. Staff may be assigned to monitor a specific exit.
- **Combative person** – a team may be assembled to present a show of force
- **Fire** – often identified as Code Red. Know the nearest exit and route.

Pharmacy Law and Regulations

HIPAA

The **Health Insurance Portability and Accountability Act** (HIPAA) enacted in 1996 went into effect in 2003. The purpose of the act is to protect patient's medical information from improper distribution while at the same time allowing for distribution under certain circumstances. HIPAA policies require healthcare professionals to do the following:

- Employ a designated privacy officer
- Devise a system to properly secure protected information
- Establish HIPAA-compliant privacy policies
- Advise patients of their rights under HIPAA and how to request their own health information
- Advise patients on how to file a complaint in the event their privacy is violated
- Train employees how to properly maintain patient privacy
- Sanction employees who do not properly follow HIPAA policies and procedures

Preparing Medications

Confidentiality is one of the top priorities in patient care. As you are preparing medications, you may be discussing the medications or providing the pharmacist with additional information about the patient. Even though the layout of the pharmacy may not provide you with a view of the patients in the waiting room, chances are good that they can still hear what you are saying. Discussing patient and prescription information loudly in a setting where other people can hear is not only a violation of trust and potentially a source of embarrassment for the patient; it is also a serious violation of HIPAA.

Patient Identifiable Information

Patient identifiable information is any information that may be used to identify a patient. This can include:

- Name
- Patient ID number
- Address
- Phone number
- Social security number

All discussion that includes patient identifiable information must take place in the most **private** setting possible. Paperwork containing this information must be kept out of sight of other patients or people who have no legitimate reason to see it. Computers containing this information must be password protected and turned in such a way so that they are not visible to other patients or the public.

Releasing Confidential Patient Information

Confidential patient information may be **released** under the following circumstances:

- To other providers who are involved in the patient's treatment in order to properly coordinate patient care
- To other parties, medical and otherwise, when accompanied by a release of information signed by the patient
- To a third party payer in order to receive correct payment
- When requested by the patient for his or her own use through a signed release of information
- To public health officials when the information poses a threat to public health, such as in case of certain infectious diseases or dog bites
- By subpoena in certain circumstances

The Joint Commission

The Joint Commission is a nonprofit, independent organization that **certifies** and **accredits** health care organizations such as hospitals throughout the United States. The Joint Commission (TJC) was formerly known as the Joint Commission on the Accreditation of Healthcare Organizations (JCAHO). Joint Commission accreditation is recognized throughout the U.S. as the **standard for best care.** The goal of The Joint Commission is to ensure the best possible healthcare for all patients at all facilities, nationwide. This is achieved by regular **inspections** of healthcare facilities, including the pharmacies. Facilities who fail to meet standards set by The Joint Commission must comply with the recommendations given within a specified timeframe and be reassessed.

FDA

The FDA is the **Food and Drug Administration**, the agency formed in 1927 to oversee the production and safety of food and drugs in the United States. The purpose of the FDA is to protect and promote public health by both supervising and regulating the production of the following:

- Food products
- Prescription medications
- Over-the-counter medications
- Tobacco products
- Dietary supplements
- Vaccines
- Biological drug products
- Blood transfusions
- Medical devices
- Cosmetics

The director of the FDA is the **Commissioner of Food and Drugs**, who is appointed by the President. The FDA also investigates and enforces laws related to food and drug safety through the **Office of Criminal Investigations**. Most of the laws that concern and affect the operation of the FDA are found in the **Food, Drug and Cosmetic Act**.

Federal Food, Drug, and Cosmetic Act

The **Federal Food, Drug, and Cosmetic Act**, often abbreviated as FD&C, gave the Food and Drug Administration oversight of the safety of the food, drug, and cosmetics industries. The FD&C Act has 20 chapters, which include sections on:

- Definitions
- Prohibitions and penalties
- Food adulteration, including bottled water
- Drugs, including homeopathic preparations
- Medical devices
- Cosmetics
- Imports and Exports

The FD&C Act went into effect in 1938 as the result of an incident in which over 100 people died after taking a medication that contained traces of diethylene glycol. Over the years, the Act has been amended multiple times, to keep up with changing technologies.

DEA

The DEA is the **Drug Enforcement Administration**, an agency of the government set up in 1973. Its purpose is to enforce laws relating to drug use, according to the Controlled Substances Act, as well as to combat drug smuggling. The DEA often shares jurisdiction with Immigrations and Customs Enforcement as well as the Federal Bureau of Investigation. The main goals of the DEA are to:

- Educate the public through youth and community-based programs to help reduce the demand for illegal and diverted drugs
- Fund state and local law enforcement to help reduce drug-related crime and violence
- Break up sources and suppliers of illegal and diverted drugs, both local and foreign

Controlled Substances Act

The Controlled Substances Act went into effect in 1970. It was approved by the U.S. Congress as Title II of the Comprehensive Drug Abuse Prevention and Control Act. All Federal laws, pertaining to the manufacture, regulation, and sale of certain controlled substances, including narcotics, were created under this policy. The five **controlled drug classes** (Schedules I – V) were created under this Act, as well as the qualifications that determined the medications that would be placed and controlled under each one. The Act, including the drug schedules, is not static, and updates are made and changed continuously to keep up with current information and research.

Prescription Drug Marketing Act

The Prescription Drug Marketing Act was signed into law in 1988. The purpose of the Act was twofold:

- To make sure that all drugs being marketed to consumers were both safe and effective
- To prevent risk to consumers from counterfeit, misbranded, adulterated, expired or subpotent medication

The Act was modified in 1992 by the **Prescription Drug Amendments**. Prior to the enactment of the Prescription Drug Marketing Act, problems with medication safety and efficacy were being reported on a regular basis. Diversion of medication was creating a major problem, with medications being sold that were unintended for transfer, including pharmaceutical samples and drugs that had been previously exported.

USP-NF

The **United States Pharmacopeia and National Formulary** are published together in a format called the USP-NF. All medication sold in the United States, both prescription and over-the-counter must comply with the standards that are set in the USP-NF. In addition to providing regulations and standards for **medication**, the USP also sets standards for **food products** and **dietary supplements**. Information about medications, including aspects of drug use, is developed by the USP and is passed down to those who make healthcare decisions, such as practitioners and pharmacists. One example of this is the system that is used by the Medicare Prescription Drug Benefit plans to create formularies. Many other countries have chosen to adopt the US's USP rather than enacting their own.

U.S. NRC

The **United States Nuclear Regulatory Committee** was created in 1975. The primary purpose of the U.S. NRC is to create standards to provide safety from **radiation**. Along with creating standards relating to issues such as nuclear reactor safety and the disposal of radioactive waste, the NRC also has responsibilities in the field of **nuclear medicine**. The NRC ensures that patients will receive the correct and proper dose of radiation as required to treat the condition, and ensures that radioactive substances used in nuclear medication are properly controlled, stored, and disposed of following use. The NRC also oversees training of pharmacists and technicians who work with nuclear medication.

Americans with Disabilities Act

The Americans with Disabilities Act (ADA) went into effect in 1990. The Act prohibits discrimination against people with disabilities. This includes discrimination in employment, public transportation, accommodations, and more. This Act requires public and commercial areas to provide **accommodations** so that people with disabilities are able to enjoy goods, services, and facilities in the same manner as fully abled people. This includes places of lodging, recreation, education, dining, transportation, stores, and health care providers. Disabilities covered are defined by the ADA as those that "substantially limit a major life activity."

Poison Prevention Packaging Act

The Poison Prevention Packaging Act went into effect in 1970. Prior to the act, **household poisonings** were one of the leading causes of death in young children. The Act was created to help fight and reduce these poisonings. The Act empowered the Consumer Products Safety Commission to set rules about packaging that would be used in households with small children. The primary result of the PPPA was creation and enforcement of the use of **child-resistant caps**. Caps are tested regularly to ensure that they meet the standards required to keep children safe.

Consumer Products Safety Commission

The Consumer Products Safety Commission, or CPSC, was created by the passage of the Consumer Products Safety Act in 1970. The purpose of the agency is to protect the public from unnecessary risks associated with **manufactured products**. The CPSC does not regulate drugs, but the **containers** in which medications are sold do fall under this agency's jurisdiction (including child resistant caps). The CPSC conducts research on products that may be considered worrisome, especially as warranted by consumer complaints, issues recalls when necessary or bans products that are considered dangerous. Consumers may lodge complaints against potentially dangerous products via the agency's toll free number or website.

Orange Book

The full title of the "Orange Book" is *Approved Drug Products with Therapeutic Equivalence and Evaluations*. A copy of this book should be available in every pharmacy, although today the Orange Book is also available online at the FDA's website. All products that have been approved by the FDA based on their proven safety and efficacy are included in the Orange Book. Medications from prior to 1938 are not included in the book. Medications are identified in the book by:

- Active ingredient
- Proprietary name
- Applicant
- Application number

The Orange Book was first published in print in 1980.

CDC

The CDC stands for the **Centers of Disease Control and Prevention**. The CDC is a government agency founded during World War II to help prevent and control the spread of communicable diseases. The purpose of the CDC is to **educate** and **inform** the public in order to improve their decisions regarding their health. They work together with local health agencies in order to get the information out to the largest number of people possible. In addition to communicable disease, the CDC also studies public health risks such as chronic diseases, disabilities, workplace health issues, environmental health issues, obesity, birth defects, and bioterrorism.

Compounding and Manufacturing Medications

The FDA defines **compounding** as preparing patient specific doses of medications as prescribed by a physician, whereas **manufacturing** is the bulk mixing or preparation of non-patient specific medications. Federal laws allow for compounding to take place on the premises of pharmacies, but not manufacture. Pharmacies violate the law allowing compounding when they:

- Compound drugs ahead of time in anticipation of prescriptions
- Compound drugs from ingredients that have been withdrawn from market
- Compound drugs from ingredients not approved by the FDA
- Compound drugs using commercial scale manufacturing or testing equipment
- Compound drugs for third-party resale
- Compound drug that are otherwise commercially available

FDA Process of Drug Approval

Drug approval is a lengthy process taking, on average, about twelve years. A drug created by a company is tested in-house for nearly four years before an application is sent to the FDA to begin the process of human testing. After the FDA approves testing, the drug enters the **three phases of human testing**:

- **Phase one** takes about a year and requires 80 to 100 healthy volunteers. Safety of the drug is tested during this time.
- **Phase two** takes approximately two years and requires 100 to 300 patient volunteers. The goal of phase two is to test efficacy of the drug.
- **Phase three** takes around three years. During this time, about 1000 to 3000 patients in hospitals and clinics will take the medication as part of the testing process while efficacy and adverse effects are carefully studied.

After testing is complete, an application is sent to the FDA for review. Once the FDA approves the new medication, it becomes available for prescription by doctors.

Recording of Distributed Prescription Medications and Controlled Substances

Pharmacies are required to keep a **log** or other file of prescriptions that have been dispensed. The prescription must be kept on file for a minimum of **five years**. The log or file must be available for inspection by the board of pharmacy and other appropriate authorities at any time. Records of dispensed medications must contain the following information:

- Date dispensed
- Drug name, strength, and dosage form
- Patient's name
- Quantity dispensed
- Patient's address

When filing prescriptions that have been filled, **CII medications** should have their own file, **CIII – CV prescriptions** should have their own file, and **other** prescription medications should have their own file.

DEA Controlled Substances

- **CI** – These substances have no recognized medical purpose, high potential for abuse, and a lack of demonstrated safety, even under medical supervision. Examples include heroin and LSD.
- **CII** – These substances have accepted medical uses (although they may have severe restrictions) and high abuse potential. Abuse may lead to physical or psychological dependence. Examples include oxycodone and methadone.
- **CIII** – Abuse potential exists, but it is lower than the potential found in CI and CII substances. These substances have accepted medical uses. Physical or psychological dependency is possible. Examples include ketamine and codeine.
- **CIV** – Abuse potential exists, but it is lower than that of CIII substances. These substances have accepted medical uses. Limited physical or psychological dependence is possible. Examples include diazepam and zolpidem.
- **CV** – These substances have a low abuse potential. These substances have an accepted medical use. Limited physical or psychological dependence is possible. Examples include pregabalin and small amounts of codeine when used in cough suppressants.

Valid Controlled Substances Prescription

A valid and legal prescription for controlled substances requires all of the following:

- Patient's full name and address
- Date written
- Prescriber's name, address, and DEA number
- Drug name, dosage form, and strength
- Prescribed quantity
- Directions for use
- Refills authorized, if any
- Handwritten signature of the prescriber (or e-signature if transmitted electronically)

If a prescription comes into the pharmacy with any of this information missing, the pharmacist must contact the **prescriber** to clarify the information. A prescriber can give verbal approval over the phone for a missing signature unless the prescription is for a controlled substance. In this case, the prescription must be returned for a physical signature.

CII Medication Faxed or Ordered Verbally

For a CII prescription to be eligible to be **faxed**, the patient must be one of the following:

- A resident in a long-term care facility
- A resident in community-based care
- Enrolled as a patient in a hospice program
- The recipient of compounded home infusion or IV pain therapy

The fax must bear the signature of the prescriber. The fax will serve as the **written prescription document**.

Verbal orders for CII prescriptions are only accepted in **emergency situations**. The amount of medication to be dispensed is limited to the amount required during the emergency period. A written prescription for the emergency quantity must be written by the prescriber and mailed or delivered to the pharmacy within seven days.

Maintaining Inventory of CII Medications

CII medications are required to be stored in a locked storage area separate from other medications, including CIII – CV medications. A perpetual **inventory** must be kept of CII medications, in which each pill dispensed is tracked manually in a **log**. The perpetual inventory must be compared and reconciled with the pharmacy's computerized inventory system on a quarterly basis. Additionally, prescriptions of CII medications must be filled separately from other prescriptions. It is never appropriate to leave CII medications out of the locked security cabinet. Many hospitals have a full room dedicated to narcotics and all orders are prepared within the narcotic room.

Changes to a CII Prescription

Before making **changes** to a CII prescription, the pharmacist is required to contact the prescriber. Only a pharmacist may take these changes from the prescriber:

- Dosage form, for example capsule vs. tablet
- Strength of the medication
- Quantity of the medication
- Directions

Even with a phone call to the doctor, the following changes are **not permitted**:

- Changes to the patient's name
- Change to a different controlled substance
- Addition of the prescriber's signature, if it was forgotten

If these changes are necessary, the patient must take the prescription back to the prescriber for a new and correct prescription.

CII Medications Transferred

To order CII medications from a wholesale warehouse, the pharmacy must properly fill out the **DEA Form 222**, either on paper or electronically. Electronic forms must be stored in such a way that they are accessible for **inspection** if required. The DEA Form 222 must contain the date and the medications ordered, as well as the quantity. The pharmacy is also required to use the DEA Form 222 to **transfer** CII medications between locations or to **return** CII medications to the wholesaler.

The following rules regarding DEA Form 222 must be followed:

- Alterations cannot be made to the form. If an error is made, the person filling it out must begin with a new form.
- The green copy of the DEA Form 222 is sent to the local DEA office.
- The blue copy of the form must be retained and kept on file at the pharmacy for at least two years.

Prescriptions Expiration and Refills

Medications that fall under CII classification are not eligible for refills. They are considered not to have an **expiration date**. It is up to the pharmacist to use his or her professional judgment in determining if the prescription should be filled. Medications that fall under CIII through CV classification are allowed up to five refills. The prescription expires six months after the date written or after five refills have been dispensed, whichever is sooner. Medications that are not scheduled may have **unlimited** (or **PRN**) refills. The prescription expires one year after the date it was written.

DEA Numbers

DEA numbers follow a very specific formula. To test the validity of a DEA number, make sure that it follows this pattern:

- DEA numbers consist of two letters followed by 6 numbers and a "check" digit.
- The first letter in the DEA number identifies the type of practitioner. For example, B indicates a hospital or clinic provider, C is a practitioner, and E is for a manufacturer.
- Add the first, third and fifth digit. This is sum A.
- Add the second, fourth and sixth digit, and multiply that answer by two. This is sum B.
- Add Sum A and Sum B.
- The last digit in your answer should be the same as the check digit at the end of the DEA number.

Restricted Drug Distribution Programs

1. **Thalidomide** uses the program **S.T.E.P.S.** (System for Thalidomide Education and Prescribing Safety). Patients are required to register, undergo pregnancy testing (if applicable), and receive mandatory counseling before receiving their first prescription. Applicable patients must undergo regularly scheduled pregnancy testing as well as mandatory counseling before subsequent prescriptions will be dispensed.
2. **Isotretinoin** uses the **iPledge program** to restrict drug distribution. Before receiving the first prescription, patients must register with the program, undergo pregnancy testing (if applicable), commit to choosing two forms of birth control, and commit to keeping all appointments as scheduled. Before receiving subsequent prescriptions, female patients must undergo monthly pregnancy tests, access the iPledge system to describe her birth control methods, and answer questions about the program.
3. **Clozapine** prescriptions require the use of a program to track the patient's **white blood cell count** as well as his or her **absolute neutrophil count**. Different manufacturers have their own programs, and any of these are acceptable as long as they allow the prescriber and pharmacist to monitor the patient's reactions to the medication.

Drug Diversion

Drug diversion is a serious problem in the health care system. Drug diversion is the use of medication for anything other than its intended purpose. It can happen at a number of different levels:

- Health care practitioners may divert drugs from stock for their own use.
- Patients may seek medications and then sell them to others.
- People may steal medications from the person to whom it was prescribed.

All of these are examples of drug diversion. Many precautions are taken at the pharmacy level to prevent drug diversion, from requiring identification to double counting-controlled medications to keeping a perpetual CII inventory log. The medications that are most commonly diverted include **opiates** such as oxycodone and hydrocodone, **stimulants** such as methylphenidate, and **depressants** such as diazepam and lorazepam. In many locations, **pseudoephedrine** is also a commonly diverted medication because it is used to make methamphetamine.

Forged Prescription

Often when drug seekers **forge** or alter prescriptions, they do so imperfectly, and it is often easy to detect. When taking in prescriptions, always check for these common "tells":

- The drug seeker may provide personal information that is contradictory.
- The prescription may be written on a form from a doctor who would not normally prescribe this type of medication, i.e. cardiologists or other specialists. This may indicate stolen prescription blanks.
- Errors made with "sig" abbreviations are often a "tell", for example, a medication that clearly does not match the usual dose (i.e. OxyContin q4h instead of bid) or simply errors using the codes (1 qbid).
- Errors in dosing may appear.
- Obvious erasures of quantities or refills can be a giveaway. Always confirm a prescription that appears to have been altered by erasing.
- Two different types of ink may indicate changes made to an otherwise valid prescription.
- Refills on CII medications can be giveaways, but may also be prescriber error. Confirm with the prescriber.
- Watch quantity numbers carefully.

Mailing a Prescription

Some pharmacies perform the service of **mailing prescriptions** to patients. Which medications can be mailed vary from state to state, so consult **local laws** before mailing medications. Prescriptions should be mailed in a special padded envelope. Packing the pill bottle with cotton will help keep tablets safe and minimize the chance of breakage. If the pharmacy you are working in is not a mail-order pharmacy and the pills are being mailed as a courtesy to the customer, notify the customer that the pills are being mailed to prevent missing medications or another miscommunication.

FDA Recall Classes I, II, and III

The FDA uses a three-class system to identify the seriousness of drug recalls.

- **Class I** recalls are the most serious. Drugs affected by a class I recall are likely to cause serious adverse health conditions or death.
- **Class II** recalls are slightly less serious. While the possibilities of death or serious health consequences are unlikely, temporary health problems may occur because of taking the drug.
- **Class III** recalls are used when a drug has violated an FDA regulation, but adverse health consequences are unlikely to occur.

Other recall actions that may occur are **FDA Market Withdrawals** in which a minor violation occurs, and either, the issue must be corrected, or the product must be withdrawn from market.

Medical devices are subject to recalls called **FDA Medical Device Safety Alerts**.

Disposing of Medications

The FDA has the following recommendations as to proper **disposal of medications**:

- Do not flush medications down the toilet unless the package specifically indicates to do so.
- If community take-back programs are offered in your area, take advantage of them.
- Before disposing of medications in the trash, medications should:
- Be removed from original containers and mixed with a substance such as used coffee grounds or cat litter, and
- Be placed in a sealed bag or other empty container to prevent leakage.
- Before disposing of a medication container, destroy the label or make it unreadable.

Ask a pharmacist for further information about proper drug disposal.

DEA Take-Back Program

The DEA Take-Back Program is a national event in which pharmacies, community partners, and law enforcement agencies are encouraged to host **collections sites** where consumers can bring back expired or other unneeded medications for safe disposal. Once the medications are collected, a local DEA representative picks them up for disposal. The goal of the National Take-Back program is to reduce the availability of drugs that could potentially be diverted and to improve consumer safety by preventing the consumption of expired medication. Additionally, Take-Back days prevent medications from being improperly disposed of and contributing to environmental contamination.

General Duties of a Certified Pharmacy Technician

Certified pharmacy technicians are responsible for many of the duties in the retail pharmacy. Some of the duties include:

- Receiving prescription orders from patients
- Checking the fax or electronic system for prescription orders
- Processing orders using pharmacy software
- Selecting correct products and counting or pouring medications to prepare the order
- Printing and attaching prescription labels
- Maintaining patient profiles
- Filing insurance claims and following up on ongoing insurance issues
- Completing transactions at the cash register

- Answering phones
- Maintaining stock and inventory in the pharmacy

Pharmacy technicians may **not** provide **medical advice** to patients. They should maintain knowledge of medications and healthcare information and be on alert for potential errors and other problems so that they can alert the pharmacist.

PHARMACY WORK ENVIRONMENTS

Pharmacy technicians are employed in a variety of pharmacy settings. Some of the places that employ certified pharmacy technicians include:

- Retail pharmacy stores
- Hospitals
- Long-term care facilities
- Mail order pharmacies
- Medical supply stores

Pharmacy technicians may work **varying hours** depending on the employer. While some technicians may work 9 to 5 shifts Monday through Friday, some retail pharmacies are open 24 hours a day and hospital pharmacies are also open around the clock. Pharmacy technicians are usually required to be available to work weekends and holidays as needed. Many pharmacy technicians also belong to professional **unions**.

RATIO OF PHARMACY TECHNICIANS TO PHARMACISTS

State laws vary on the exact **ratio** of technicians to pharmacists allowed at a given time. Some states offer a suggested ratio, while others define the number as a law. Some states require a 2:1 ratio, while others allow for a 3:1 ratio. The purpose of keeping the ratio of techs to pharmacists low is to allow the pharmacist to provide adequate **supervision** of the technicians under his or her authority. If there are too many technicians and not enough pharmacists, it is difficult to guarantee that prescriptions and prepared medications are being fully checked before being dispensed.

GENERAL DUTIES OF A CERTIFIED PHARMACY TECHNICIAN IN A HOSPITAL

In a hospital setting, pharmacy technician duties are likely to include the following:

- Maintenance of stock, including ordering stock, putting away inventory, pulling expired stock, and preparing returns
- Tracking and maintaining narcotic inventory
- Preparing IV and other sterile admixture, including chemotherapy and parenteral nutrition, under the supervision of a pharmacist
- Selecting the correct medication to fill orders
- Preparing medication for dispensing throughout the hospital
- Checking other technicians' work, depending on local laws
- Delivering medication throughout the hospital to units and nursing floors on both a scheduled basis and an as-needed basis
- Maintaining medication delivery systems, such as automated dispensing devices
- Updating and maintaining patient profiles
- Maintaining the cleanliness of the pharmacy
- Assisting with the training of new technicians

Dispensing of Medication

In most hospitals, the **nursing station** is the hub of each section. It is where the nurses come to get information and instructions for their day. Often, **automatic dispensing devices** are located at the nursing station. If the hospital uses a pneumatic tube system, each nurses' station is likely to have a **tube stop**. The pharmacy technician loads the dispensing device or sends individual doses through the tubes. Nurses remove the medications and dispense them according to physician instructions. It is important for nurses to follow the same rules about medication storage as the pharmacy. Occasionally, training is given to ensure that rules are being followed uniformly throughout the hospital. Pharmacy technicians may be sent to inspect the area to make sure that medications are stored according to law and hospital policy.

Dress Codes for Technicians

Many pharmacies require specific **dress codes** for pharmacy technicians. While retail pharmacies often require business casual clothing for a professional appearance, hospital pharmacies often establish dress codes with safety and cleanliness in mind. Depending on the area of the pharmacy where the technician works, any of the following might be required:

- Scrubs
- Foot covers
- Hair bonnets
- Masks
- Goggles or other eye coverings

Shoes in the pharmacy are required to be **closed toe**. Not only is this for sanitary purposes, it is also an important safety measure, especially when working with needles and syringes, which can fall out of hands.

Cleaning Items Used to Count Medication

As work proceeds in the pharmacy, items used to measure, count, and pour medication may become dirty or **contaminated** with dust from the medications. It is important to wash counting trays and spatulas as well as other measurement tools at least once a day with hot soapy water. Throughout the day, keep cleaning wipes available to wipe down counting trays on a regular basis. It is especially important to wipe trays and spatulas down after counting out pills of medications that are known to frequently cause allergies, such as **penicillin** or **sulfa antibiotics.** Powder from these medications could contaminate other medications counted on the same equipment and cause an allergic reaction. Many pharmacies have separate counting trays specifically for these medications for this reason. Immediately clean tools used to pour or scoop liquid and cream medications after use.

Areas of the Pharmacy to Be Cleaned Every Day

One of the duties of a pharmacy technician is to maintain the **cleanliness** of the pharmacy. The pharmacy should be as clean as possible. **Dusting** should be done on a regular basis. Daily cleaning duties include:

- Wiping down the counter and all surface areas
- Cleaning all tools used to dispense medications
- Wiping down keyboards and all phone surfaces
- Removing trash from the pharmacy
- Sweeping or vacuuming the floor of the pharmacy

- Wet-mopping the floor of the pharmacy with disinfectant
- Clean the seating in the lobby or waiting area with disinfectant, also the area should be swept and wet-mopped with disinfectant or vacuumed.

Preceptor

Pharmacy preceptors are teachers and mentors to pharmacy trainees. Before a pharmacy can take on interns or other trainees, the pharmacist must train and apply for **preceptor certification**. While preceptor requirements vary depending on local laws, generally the following is required:

- One to two years of full-time employment as a pharmacist at the location where they plan to be a preceptor
- Fully licensed and maintaining good standing with the local Board of Pharmacy
- Willingness and desire to mentor students
- Willingness and desire to perform honest assessments of the students' abilities
- Willingness to have their performance as a preceptor assessed by students

State Board of Pharmacy

Each state has its own board of pharmacy. The board of pharmacy licenses pharmacies, pharmacists, and technicians as part of the state's **department of health**. Other specific functions may vary from state to state. The ultimate goal is to promote public health and safety by ensuring that every pharmacy in the state is operating under the same set of high standards. The board of pharmacy also works as a go-between to ease communication between the public, pharmacies, and state governmental agencies. The state board of pharmacy **inspects** and **grades** pharmacies to ensure they are meeting the set standards.

NABP

The NABP is the **National Association of the Boards of Pharmacy**. The purpose of the organization is to assist and support the individual state boards of pharmacy. They are intended to remain impartial and to help keep standards as uniform as possible across the states. The NABP also helps facilitate the transfer of pharmacist licenses across state lines. The organization was founded in 1904. As well as helping to maintain pharmacy standards, the NABP also provides examinations to assess pharmacist competence. The ultimate goal of the NABP is to promote and protect public safety.

SDS

SDS (formerly MSDS) stands for **Safety Data Sheets**. These pages (also available online with a subscription) provide information about the following materials and chemical compounds, including physical features and proper procedures and precautions to take in case of a spill. Every pharmacy should have an **SDS book** (or online access) that is easily accessible in the case of an accident. This is an **OSHA requirement**. Specific information listed on SDS includes:

- Manufacturer
- Contractor information
- Identified hazards based on routes of entry
- Potential for carcinogenicity or other hazards
- Potential for fire hazard or explosion and methods for extinguishing if flammable
- First aid treatment
- Clean up requirements

- Recommended safety equipment
- Directions for disposal

Chemical Spill

In the event of a chemical spill, follow the detailed **spill response plan** located in the pharmacy. The plan will generally follow these steps:

- Immediately warn everyone in the area of the spill, and evacuate if necessary.
- Remove contaminated clothing, and flush skin that has come into contact with the chemical.
- Refer to the Safety Data Sheet to get more information about the spilled chemical, including flammability and volatility.
- Don personal protective equipment, including respiratory protection, if needed.
- For small or medium spills, use the absorption spill kit. You should know the location of this kit in your pharmacy.
- For large spills, outside help may be required. Follow local procedures and policies.
- Once the spill has been absorbed, dispose of it in appropriate chemical spill bags.
- Decontaminate the area with water and detergent when appropriate.
- Report spills to supervisor.

Hazardous Waste

Pharmacies can produce quite a bit of **hazardous waste**. Hazardous waste in the pharmacy includes all of the following:

- Expired medications
- Medications that have been incorrectly compounded
- Chemotherapy
- Products contaminated with bodily fluids
- Items used to dispense or compound hazardous materials

An outside company often picks up **pharmaceutical waste**. To prepare waste for pickup, items should be placed in bags marked with the hazardous or biohazard logo to identify them. A bin that is specifically designed for hazardous waste collection should be used to store the waste until it can be picked up.

Eye Irrigation Station

In case of medication or other chemicals accidentally splashing into the eye, use the **eye irrigation station** as follows:

- If wearing contact lenses, remove immediately.
- Hold the eyes open and position face so that eyes are properly placed.
- Have someone assist you with turning on the station. Someone else should call for emergency assistance.
- Allow water to flush continuously over the eyes until substance is removed (at least 15 minutes).

Some locations may not have an emergency eyewash station. In this situation, flush the eyes with normal **saline** and be seen by an emergency medical provider immediately.

Accidental Skin Contact with a Hazardous Substance

Skin contact with a medication or chemical in the pharmacy is a possibility. **Accidental exposure** could result in burns, blisters, rash, hives, irritation, or reddening of the skin. If exposure occurs, notify a supervisor immediately. Remove any contaminated clothing. Run cool water over the affected area for at least 15 minutes. If the area is painful, apply cool, wet compresses. However, if a burn has occurred, cover the area with dry sterile dressing. If a second or third degree burn has occurred, get medical help immediately. The best way to prevent accidental contact with hazardous substances is the consistent use of **personal protective equipment**, such as gloves or gowns.

Ingestion of a Hazardous Substance

Ingestion of hazardous substances or poisoning is treated according to the substance that has been ingested.

- Notify a supervisor immediately.
- Identify the substance. Locate the SDS for the substance and find the information on treatment.
- If indicated, induce vomiting with a product like ipecac syrup, however, if the substance is corrosive or if the victim is unconscious, do not induce vomiting.
- Call for emergency medical assistance immediately.

To prevent accidental ingestion, keep food items well away from medication preparation areas in the pharmacy and never store foods in a refrigerator or freezer intended for drug storage. Additionally, wearing a **facemask** while preparing or compounding medications will also prevent accidents from occurring.

Inhalation of a Hazardous Substance

Inhalation of hazardous material can occur in the pharmacy when working with powders used for compounding or the preparation of IV medications. In the case of an accidental inhalation, the following steps should occur:

- Notify a supervisor immediately.
- Evacuate into fresh air.
- Make sure the person who inhaled the chemicals can still breathe.
- Call for emergency medical assistance.

Inhalation of chemicals and hazardous substances can be prevented by using **personal protective equipment** such as a mask when preparing a compound using a powder. Good **airflow** can prevent a spill from contaminating the entire pharmacy, although the area should still be evacuated until it is declared safe.

First, Second, and Third-Degree Burns

Burns are classified as first, second, or third degree according to their severity based on damage to the tissue.

- **First-degree burns** are the least serious. The skin may become red, swollen, and painful, but the outer layer of skin is still intact. First aid includes running cool water over the area for 10 to 15 minutes or covering with cool compresses.

- In a **second-degree burn**, the outer layer of skin is damaged. Blisters result, and there may be severe pain and swelling. A small second-degree burn can be treated like a first-degree burn. A large second-degree burn or one on the hands, feet, face, or major joint requires immediate medical assistance.
- **Third-degree burns** are extremely serious. The skin and underlying tissue are burned through. There may be charring, or the area may look white and dry. Call 911 immediately for a third-degree burn. If possible, elevate the burned area above the heart, and cover with cool, moist, sterile bandages.

Continuing Education

Continuing education booklets, articles, and tests can be found in a number of places. Some pharmacy associations hold seminars and classes that technicians can attend for **CE credits**. Numerous pharmacy publications contain articles that are worth CE credits. Many websites also offer CE, including the PTCB website, Powerpak.com, Freece.com, and rxschool.com. Track CE credits carefully, and keep printouts of completed CE credits to demonstrate compliance, if necessary. Twenty contact hours are necessary to **recertify**, with at least one of those hours in **pharmacy law**. Up to ten hours may be earned under the supervision of your pharmacist, but it must be in an area that is not included in your daily duties. One college course can qualify as 15 continuing education credits during each two-year period.

Updates on Pharmacy Law

State and federal pharmacy laws are updated frequently. Technicians can check the following sources for the most current pharmacy law information:

- The **Drug Enforcement Administration** website, available at www.dea.gov
- The website for their own state's board of pharmacy
- The **National Pharmacy Technician Association** website and newsletter, available at www.pharmacytechnician.org
- **Pharmacy magazines** including Drug Topics, Rx Times, U.S. Pharmacist, and Pharmacy Times

Not only is it important to stay on top of changes in law from a personal and professional standpoint, one of a certified pharmacy technician's twenty **continuing education hours** must be in law to keep certification current. Check continuing education sources for modules related to pharmacy law.

Sterile and Non-Sterile Compounding

Compounded Medication

A compounded medication is any medication that is created by a pharmacist or a technician in order to meet specific dosing requirements given by the prescriber. Compounding can include changing a drug's **dosage form**, for example from a powder to a cream or from a capsule to a suspension. Compounding also includes the preparation of individualized **injectable medications**. Typically, compounding is done in order to meet specific and unique needs of a patient, for example, a patient unable to take pills, or to create a dose otherwise unavailable for an infant. Some compounding, such as adding flavor to a medication, is done optionally to improve **compliance**.

Compounding

Properly compounding a medication requires the following steps:

- Entering the prescription into the pharmacy software as directed (some pharmacies have a separate software system specifically for prescriptions requiring compounding)
- Preparing the compounding area, including cleaning and laying out compounding paper
- Assembling the correct medications, inert ingredients, and compounding supplies
- Calibrating the equipment
- Performing the calculations or double checking calculations that have been provided
- Compounding the medications, using aseptic technique if compounding sterile products
- Recording the expiration dates of the compounded medications
- Preparing the order for check by the pharmacist, this includes keeping all packaging of equipment and the original packaging of the compounded ingredients.

Compounding Equipment and Supplies

The equipment and supplies that should be gathered prior to compounding a **cream** or **ointment** include:

- A Class A prescription balance or analytical balance to weigh out the ingredients
- Weighing papers, for use with the balance
- A spatula to transfer ingredients such as the base to the weighing paper or pans
- A mortar and pestle if particles need to be reduced to a fine powder
- A graduate if liquids will be incorporated in the compound
- An ointment slab
- The medication to be compounded
- The cream or ointment base
- Wetting agent or levigating agent, if necessary

Equipment Required to Compound a Sterile Product

To compound a **sterile product** in a clean environment, the following supplies should be gathered before beginning:

- Personal protective equipment, such as gloves, gown, hair bonnet, mask, and foot coverings, if necessary
- Sterile admixture should always be done under a laminar flow hood that has been cleaned in the correct fashion
- Vials or ampules of medication to be compounded

- Appropriately sized syringes
- Filter needles if drawing from an ampule
- IV bags or solutions into which the medication will be mixed
- Alcohol for cleaning the hood
- Alcohol wipes for disinfecting rubber stoppers prior to inserting a needle

Checking a Compounded Medication

Before the pharmacist can **check** a compounded medication prepared by a technician; the following should be gathered for the pharmacist to inspect:

- The original order and prescription label
- The calculations made to determine the correct dose
- The vials or containers of the medications and solutions used
- If preparing an injectable, the syringe used to withdraw the medication from the vial, pulled back to the dose used
- If the medication was drawn from an ampule, the packaging from the filter needle to show that it was used
- The finished product, free of contamination and particulates

Extemporaneous Compound

An extemporaneous compound or extemporaneous prescription is one that is prepared on demand by the pharmacist or technician to meet the needs of a unique patient. The compound is created to meet specific **quantity**, **strength**, and **dosage form** needs set by the prescriber and contains pharmaceutical product. Examples of common extemporaneous compounds include creams, ointments, suspensions, and suppositories. Careful calculation and preparation technique is required to ensure that the compound contains the **exact amount** of medication required and is prepared in a sanitary fashion to avoid introducing **contaminants** into the compound.

Aseptic Technique

Aseptic technique is used to prepare IV admixtures and other sterile products. It ensures that the products remain **sterile** during preparation. Poor technique is a serious risk to patients. Aseptic technique should always be done in a **laminar flow hood**. Always maintain space between the HEPA filter and the product being mixed. The airflow is what keeps the mixture and supplies free of particulates. Possible obstructions include hands, IV bags, and other equipment. When drawing product from a syringe or ampule, be careful not to touch the plunger anywhere except on the back. Complete calculations before entering the hood, and do not allow clutter in the hood. Remove jewelry from hands and arms and wash hands and arms before entering the hood. Keep hands in the hood as much as possible. If you touch your face, hair, or clothing, you must wash again. Do not talk, sneeze, or cough while preparing medications in the hood. Before puncturing with a needle, wipe down all rubber stoppers with alcohol.

Preparing Sterile Products

When preparing sterile products, it is important to take the following precautions:

- Check the drug to be sure that it is within date and not otherwise compromised. A multi-use vial contains preservatives, but a single-use vial can no longer be guaranteed sterile once it has been punctured and must be discarded even if medication remains.
- Wash your hands frequently.
- Do not wear jewelry.

- Wear gloves, gown, and bonnet, if required.
- Do not speak or cough into the hood.
- Do not touch the needle or the plunger on the syringe.
- Wipe rubber stoppers with alcohol before inserting the needle.
- Know aseptic technique, and use it.
- Sanitize the preparation area thoroughly before and after use.

Medications Considered Sterile Products

The following medications are sterile products and should be prepared as such, using **aseptic technique**:

- Intravenous medications
- Total parenteral nutrition
- Intramuscular medications
- Ophthalmic solutions and suspensions
- Subcutaneous medications
- Chemotherapy

Sterile product must also be **stored** in such a way as to guarantee its sterility. Different medications have different storage requirements. Consult with your pharmacy manager to learn your storage protocol at your location. Keep the access port covered on IV bags to prevent contamination. Foil or plastic coverings are used for this. Keep this port covered until the medication is delivered to the patient or the nurse.

Contamination in Sterile Preparations

Despite best practice and aseptic technique, occasionally **contamination** may still occur. Before dispensing a sterile medication, always check for the following signs that may indicate contamination:

- Formation of precipitate
- Unidentified objects in the solutions (may indicate that coring has occurred)
- Cloudiness when the solution should be clear
- A change in color that is unanticipated
- A regular needle used to withdraw medication from a glass ampule
- Separation of the ingredients

If the solution cannot be guaranteed sterile, show the pharmacist the solution with the error in order to help prevent future errors, and remake the solution.

Proper Hand-Washing Technique

Preparation of sterile medications requires hands to be as clean as possible. The following **hand-washing technique** should be used when preparing medication in a clean room or under a laminar flow hood:

1. Remove rings, watches, and other jewelry.
2. Use a foot pedal or paper towel to turn on the faucet.
3. Wet your hands up to the forearms with warm water.
4. Apply antibacterial soap or other preparation used for disinfecting.
5. Scrub each hand for at least 30 seconds, using the fingers of the other hand.

6. Rinse thoroughly, holding the arms in a downward position so that the water runs down over the fingertips instead of down into clothing.
7. Dry your hands using a clean, sterile towel.
8. Turn off the faucet using the sterile towel and discard towel.

Laminar Flow Hood

A laminar flow hood is designed in such a way to provide a space free of contaminants and particulates for the purpose of compounding sterile preparations in the pharmacy. Air from the room is drawn through a **HEPA filter** and blown back toward the user in order to keep a steady stream of filtered air flowing over the items in the hood. Both vertical and horizontal hoods are available, as well as others with different airflow patterns designed for specific uses. The laminar flow hood must be maintained according to manufacturer specifications and cleaned thoroughly before every use to ensure no contaminants are present.

Properly Prepare and Clean the IV Admixture Hood

Cleaning the laminar flow hood requires proper technique. The steps in this technique are:

1. Collect your cleaning equipment: 70% ethanol or other disinfectant and sterile gauze or other laboratory grade wipes.
2. Dress in personal protective equipment including gloves, mask, goggles, foot coverings, and gown.
3. Turn the hood on, and allow the hood to run for five minutes. Remove any items that do not belong in the hood.
4. Spray the internal surfaces with the disinfectant, and clean with sterile wipes using a sweeping back and forth motion. Do not spray disinfectant into the HEPA filter.
5. Allow the hood to air dry.

Total Parenteral Nutrition

Total parenteral nutrition is liquid food that is administered to the patient **intravenously**. Parenteral nutrition may be done for a number of reasons. For example, the patient may have recently had surgery or may have a health condition that causes him or her to be unable take food orally. Pharmacy technicians are often called upon to mix total parenteral nutrition (TPN). **TPN** is a mixture of proteins, sugars, lipids, vitamins, and minerals — everything needed to meet nutritional needs. When preparing TPN, a pharmacy technician should do the following:

- Verify the order, and double check calculations.
- Generate labels, and verify for accuracy.
- Gather ingredients, and mix under a laminar flow hood using a compounder.
- Affix an expiration date of no later than 36 hours.
- Prepare mixture for checking by a pharmacist.

Chemical Incompatibility

Some medications are physically and chemically **incompatible** and should never be mixed. Some of the problems that may arise are:

- Formation of precipitates or crystallization
- Formation of gas or other noxious chemical compounds
- The ingredients do not mix to form a solution, for example, one floats on the other or the ingredients congeal

Examples:

- **Diazepam** dissolves poorly, which can lead to precipitates forming when improperly diluted
- Mixing **phenytoin** with 5% **glucose** solution leads to nearly immediate precipitation
- Combining **magnesium sulfate** and **calcium chloride** in the same bag will cause a precipitation of calcium sulfate

Medication Safety

Radiopharmaceuticals

A radiopharmaceutical is a substance that the patient ingests in order to help **diagnose** or **treat** certain conditions such as cancers, colorectal disease, certain bone diseases, and more. Radiopharmaceuticals may be taken orally, injected, or instilled into the eye or the bladder. Although some radioactivity is present in the agent, the amount is so small that it is not harmful to the body. Some agents may be given in larger doses when treating a disease. In this situation, the effect on the body varies. When a radiopharmaceutical is being used to diagnose a condition, the agent passes through the organ or system in question or is absorbed by it. Special visualizing equipment is then used to detect the radioactivity, and a **diagnosis** can be made based on the workings of the organ or system.

Chemotherapy

Chemotherapy or **antineoplastic drugs** are medications and combinations of medications used to treat a variety of cancers. The goal of the chemotherapy is to kill the cells that are rapidly multiplying in order to halt and reverse the growth of the **tumors**. Chemotherapy also kills off healthy cells and, as a result, has a number of unfortunate side effects including **hair loss**, **nausea**, and **immunosuppression**. Chemotherapy medications can be taken orally or infused intravenously. Often chemotherapy in combination with radiation and other treatments is used in the aggressive treatment of cancer. Some of the different types of chemotherapy include:

- Alkylating agents like cisplatin and oxaliplatin
- Antimetabolites
- Vinca alkaloids including vincristine and vinblastine
- Taxanes such as paclitaxel and docetaxel

Exposure to Chemotherapy

Unintentional exposure to chemotherapy agents is a very real risk of working in a pharmacy. Some of the ways in which this exposure may occur are:

- **Inhalation** may occur if a technician breathes in chemotherapy agents that have been aerosolized or distributed as airborne particles.
- **Absorption** may occur if unprotected skin comes into contact with the chemotherapy agent.
- **Ingestion** of the chemotherapy agent can occur from hand to mouth transmission.
- **Injection** can occur due to accidental needle sticks during the preparation of injectable chemotherapy agents.

Exposure to chemotherapy agents can cause a number of consequences, including short-term effects such as skin rashes, blistering, and irritation. Long-term consequences could be severe including miscarriages, birth defects in future children, and the development of cancer.

Chemotherapy Agent's Exposure Prevention

Pharmacies have taken a number of steps in order to **prevent** staff from exposure to chemotherapy agents. Some of these steps include:

- Biological safety cabinets or compounding aseptic containment isolators, which provide filtered air to the area and allow the air to vent out safely while a glass shield protects the operator from contact
- Negatively pressured clean rooms, which keep contaminated air from blowing into other areas
- The use of personal protective equipment such as gowns, masks, gloves, hair covers, shoe covers, and goggles
- Policies requiring frequent changes of personal protective equipment in order to prevent contamination

Drug handling techniques include the negative pressure technique to extract medications from vials to prevent aerosolization and splatter, proper ampule extraction technique, and appropriate sharps disposal.

Ear and Eye Solutions and Suspensions

Some doctors may occasionally prescribe **ocular preparations** to be used in the ear when the medication and strength is not available in an otic preparation. This is acceptable; however, otic preparations cannot be used to fill a prescription intended for ocular use. This is because otic preparations contain **preservatives** that are not intended to be used in the eyes and could cause serious side effects, including burning and itching. When filling a medication for ocular or otic use, always be careful to select the proper formulation. Notify the pharmacist in case of prescriber error. A phone call to the prescriber may be necessary.

Coring the Rubber Stopper

Unless proper syringe technique is used, part of the rubber stopper may shear off and lodge itself in the hollow needle. This is known as **coring**, and it has the potential to contaminate the medication and cause serious risks to the patient. If the coring goes unnoticed, and the core is injected into the patient, it could lead to death. To prevent coring, the needle should be introduced into the rubber stopper at a 45 to 60-degree angle, with the opening facing up and away from the stopper. As the needle is pushed into the stopper, the amount of pressure is slightly increased, as is the angle. As the needle bevel is passed through the stopper, the needle should be at a 90-degree angle or straight up.

Counseling by a Pharmacist

Every patient receiving a new prescription must be offered **counseling** by a pharmacist. This requirement is law in the majority of states. Counseling serves a number of purposes:

- It offers a final check to make sure the right patient is getting the right medication for the right condition.
- It allows the pharmacist to discuss potential side effects with the patient and offer instruction on what to do should they occur.
- It allows the pharmacist to add and emphasize special instructions such as whether or not the medication should be taken with food, or if it should be taken at a particular time of day.
- It allows the pharmacist to explain any interactions that may occur.

- It allows the pharmacist to determine the level of health literacy of the patient and adjust instruction accordingly.
- It improves patient compliance.

Common Prescription Errors

Doctors often make **errors** on prescriptions that can be easily confirmed with a phone call. Some of the most common errors include:

- Forgetting to write in the patient's name or writing the wrong name
- Date errors, including putting the wrong date or forgetting to write the date.
- Misspelled medications
- Directions that don't match the medication
- Refills on CII medications
- Forgetting to sign the prescription
- Sloppy handwriting that makes it difficult to interpret the name of the medication
- Forgetting to write the quantity or days' supply
- Writing for a dose that doesn't exist
- Simply writing "take as directed" ("Take as directed" is not a valid sig. This must be clarified to provide the correct quantity and days' supply.)
- Leaving off the route of administration when more than one is possible

Visual Impairment

Visual impairment can prove challenging for patients who are taking medications or other forms of therapy. Some of the difficulties that may arise include:

- Inability to read the directions on the bottle
- Inability to identify the medication based on the size and shape of the pill
- Inability to recognize potential mistakes made by the pharmacy (i.e. changes in the color of a medication)

Pharmacies can help improve the situation in several ways:

- Putting medications in differently sized bottles
- Providing thorough counseling and letting patients feel the shape and size of the medication so that they can easily identify it at home.
- Helping the patient or caregiver prepare a Mediset or other system for easily taking medications that doesn't require pill bottles (many of these come with Braille on the lids)
- Providing handouts in Braille

Syringes

Insulin is dosed in units, and insulin syringes reflect this, providing sizes and measurements in **units** rather than ccs or mLs. Insulin syringes are available in a variety of sizes and are tipped with various needle sizes. Needle sizes are measured in **length** and **gauge**. Most insulin syringe needles are available in 28 to 31 gauges, with a higher gauge number indicating a finer needle. The patient's personal preference often comes into play, as slightly thicker needles are less flexible and can be longer. When selecting a box of insulin needles, be careful to select a unit size as close to the patient's insulin dose as possible without going under. If the syringe is too small, the patient will have to administer two injections. If the syringe is too large, the accuracy of the dose deteriorates.

Signs of Noncompliance in Taking Medications

For medications to work properly, they must be taken **as directed**. Estimates indicated that at least 10 percent of all E.R. visits are due to patients not taking medication as directed. Many people die every year because they are not taking their prescribed medications at the correct dosages or at all. Patients who are suspected of being **noncompliant** about their medications should be pointed out to the pharmacist for additional counseling to find out what is causing the compliance problem. Some signs that identify noncompliant patients include:

- Consistently late refills
- Questions about splitting pills when the dose doesn't require it
- Dropping off multiple prescriptions but only filling one
- Phone calls from the doctor about missed appointments

Missed Dose

Always refer patients who have **missed a dose** or who have other concerns about their medication to the pharmacist for counseling. What the patient should do depends greatly on which medication was missed. Most medications require the patient to take the missed dose as soon as they realize it, or, if it is almost time for the next dose, to skip the missed dose, and take the next dose as scheduled. Other medications require the patient to take a double dose the next day. However, some medications must be taken at the scheduled time and should be skipped completely if they are missed.

Drug Stability

Drug stability is dependent on a number of different factors. Some drugs degrade faster when exposed to **light** (requiring them to be stored in opaque or darkly tinted bottles), some degrade faster when exposed to **heat** (requiring them to be refrigerated), and others degrade quickly upon exposure to **oxygen** (meaning that their expiration date, once opened, changes). For this reason, drugs that are dispensed must have an **expiration date** on the bottle no greater than one year following the dispensing date. Medications that are mixed often have a **post-mixing expiration period** printed on the bottle (for example, 10 days after mixing), and this information should be used to determine the expiration date. **Nitroglycerin tablets** begin to degrade once the sealed bottle is opened, therefore a pharmacist should counsel patients regarding the expiration date of such medications.

Epidural Administration vs. Intravenous Administration

When preparing a medication that is to be administered via epidural injection, it is crucial that the medications used do not contain **preservatives**. Medications for epidural administration must be clearly marked to prevent confusion and accidental administration of medications intended for intravenous delivery. Administering a medication that contains preservatives via epidural carries a strong risk of **neurotoxicity** and dangerous side effects, including damage to the epidural tissue and numerous neurological symptoms. Preservative-free medications and those containing preservatives should be stored separately in the pharmacy to prevent errors. Technicians performing admixture should prepare medications intended for IV use and medications intended for epidural use in separate batches to avoid mix-ups.

Extravasation

Extravasation occurs when medications intended for intravenous administration are administered into the tissue around the site rather than into the vein. This can happen in a few different ways:

- Leakage due to damaged veins. This occurs occasionally in the elderly and in people with otherwise compromised veins.
- Leaking from a hole in the vein that was created by a previous injection
- Improper technique when placing the infusion

Extravasation is a serious adverse event that can result in numerous side effects, including **tissue necrosis**. While side effects are possible with extravasation of any medication, they are particularly concerning when extravasation occurs with **chemotherapy**.

Cultural Sensitivity

Cultural sensitivity or cultural awareness is the knowledge that your customers will be from a variety of cultures, some of whom have different **experiences** and **values** when it comes to healthcare. It is important to recognize and be respectful of those differences when assisting patients. Some of the ways pharmacies can be respectful of other cultures include:

- Printing out prescription labels and counseling patients in their own language
- Asking customers questions to clarify and understand when they express a concern about the medication based on religious or cultural beliefs
- Expressing the benefits and drawbacks of medical therapy vs. alternative therapies without sounding judgmental
- Recognizing when a patient may require additional assistance even though they may not be willing to say so

Health Literacy

Health literacy is a person's ability to understand and make decisions regarding his or her healthcare. Health literacy incorporates a wide range of abilities, from a complete lack of understanding, which leads to medication mistakes, missed appointments, and noncompliance, to a thorough understanding of how insurance companies operate as well as a good grasp of the functioning of multiple systems in the body. People with **low health literacy** will require extra counseling and assistance to ensure that they are receiving proper medical care. Being aware of the potential health literacy of your patients and pointing out those that may not be as health literate to the pharmacist for extra counseling is a valuable service to those patients.

Low Health Literacy

Some of the population groups who are likely to have low health literacy and require extra assistance include:

- The elderly
- Immigrants
- Minorities
- People with lower income

While it is important to identify people with low health literacy so that they can receive additional counseling, it is also important not to resort to **stereotypes** that can be potentially insulting. For example, an elderly patient may be a retired doctor and may be offended if spoken to as if he were unaware of how his medication works. Listen carefully to your patients' speech, the questions they ask as well as the concerns they verbalize, in order to identify those who may have low health literacy.

Additional Pharmacist Counseling

While people in certain groups are more likely to have low health literacy, not all members of those groups have difficulties. It is important to identify those with challenges while not insulting others who do not. Some signs that a patient may require **extra assistance** include:

- A patient who can't identify the condition for which they have been prescribed the medication
- A patient who nods his or her head when asked a question, without actually answering
- A patient who agrees to everything but doesn't ask informed questions
- A patient who makes mistakes filling out an intake form or leaves large areas blank
- Statements such as "I will read this later" or "I forgot my glasses"

Communication with Patients

As a pharmacy technician, you can help improve care for people who have **lower health literacy** by doing the following:

- Identifying people who appear to have low health literacy and informing the pharmacist
- Listening to the concerns patients express and bringing the pharmacist over to help answer the patient's questions
- Speaking clearly without using medical jargon (for example, referring to a medication as a "blood pressure pill" instead of "antihypertensive")
- Using short sentences
- Selecting appropriate auxiliary labels
- Asking the patient questions to confirm understanding
- Have a pleasant and inviting demeanor to help the patient feel more comfortable

Patient Counseling

The pharmacist is the only person that should do **patient counseling**. In some cases, a pharmacy intern may be allowed to counsel when supervised by a preceptor. Counseling must be offered to **every patient**. The purpose is for the pharmacist to make sure the patient understands the directions, side effects, and other important information about the medication. Additional information that may be gathered during a counseling session is the condition the medication is intended to treat as well as other medications the patient is currently taking. These sessions are crucial to ensure that the patient takes the medication correctly, to improve compliance and help the patient's condition improve.

Counseling Refusal

Patients may **refuse** counseling if the medication is a refill or the patient has been taking the medication for a while (although pharmacist counseling should still be offered as the patient may still have questions or concerns). If a patient chooses to decline counseling, he or she must provide a **record** of the refusal along with a signature. This record may be kept electronically or stored in a file. The person offering the counseling should never use a voice or tone that would indicate that counseling the patient would be a bother or an inconvenience. The ultimate goal is to improve patient safety, which can be partly achieved by counseling all patients.

Unnecessary or Expired Medications

When medications that are **no longer necessary** or that are **expired** are kept around the house, the following problems could potentially occur:

- Diversion from family members or guests in the household
- Drugs may be retrieved from the trash and sold or abused
- Drugs may be found by children and ingested, leading to accidental poisonings, especially if the medications are not stored in their original containers with child-resistant caps
- Drugs may be disposed of improperly, leading to further abuse or damage to the environment
- Medications taken past their expiration date may be less effective or can even be dangerous

Child Resistant Caps

Child resistant caps, also known as child resistant packaging, are used to prevent injuries and deaths caused by children ingesting medications. The lids use a device that requires an understanding of the process and manual dexterity to open the bottles. Some require lines to be matched up, while others require the cap to be squeezed or pressed downward while opening. Child resistant caps must be used on **every prescription dispensed**. The patient does have the right to waive this requirement, usually by signing a waiver that removes responsibility from the pharmacy. Local laws and policies as to how this is handled will vary.

Child Resistant Verses Childproof Caps

When describing packaging designed to keep children from opening it, the preferred terminology is "**child resistant**." It is referred to in this way to help develop the mindset that no packaging will ever be perfectly childproof. Even packages and bottles designed to be child resistant should be kept out of the reach of children to prevent accidental poisonings and overdoses, which could be fatal. Children have been known to figure out how to open child resistant caps and packages. Packaging should never be thought of as a first line of defense.

Tetracycline

Ideally, no medication should ever be used past its expiration date, but **tetracycline** is a special case. Tetracycline drugs, like minocycline, become **toxic** after the expiration date. Chemicals in the capsules break down and can cause damage to the **kidneys** if taken past the expiration date. If a course of tetracycline is discontinued before completion per doctor's orders, the remainder of the medication should be disposed of in an appropriate manner. Do not stop taking antibiotics without the advice of a doctor or pharmacist. Discontinuing antibiotics prematurely may lead to a **recurrence** of the infection and it contributes to the increase in **drug-resistant bacteria**.

Phone Calls

As a technician, it is important to realize which phone calls are within the **technician's** scope of practice to answer and which should be given to a **pharmacist**. The technician can handle any of the following calls:

- General store information queries
- Requests for refills
- Questions regarding quantities of refills left
- Pricing questions
- Questions regarding insurance

Any phone call requiring **specialized knowledge** or **professional advice** must be passed to the pharmacist. These include:

- Questions about the actions of medications
- Questions about interactions
- Recommendations for medications or other treatment
- New prescriptions calls from doctors
- Any other questions requiring medical advice

Pharmacy Quality Assurance

Improve Quality Control and Prevent Mistakes

One of the top priorities of every pharmacy is **preventing mistakes**. Typical quality control measures include:

- Counseling every patient on the proper use of the medication
- Avoiding abbreviations and medical jargon
- Identifying "sound-alike" drugs (for example Celebrex and Celexa, Lamictal and Lamisil) and marking them in the pharmacy to increase awareness
- Identifying "high alert" medications within the pharmacy and labeling them (such as warfarin)
- Using computer software to identify potential interactions and therapeutic duplication (don't bypass checks)
- Taking the time to carefully check and double check medications and not allowing yourself to be rushed
- Reporting any errors appropriately to identify system failures and improve the process
- Keeping appropriate levels of trained staff in the pharmacy at all times

Calibration

Numerous items in the pharmacy require **calibration** to protect patient safety, ensure the integrity of medication being dispensed, and prevent incorrect dosing (over or under) from occurring. Some of the equipment in the pharmacy that should be checked and calibrated on a regular basis includes:

- Scales that are used to count medications
- Scales used to weigh ingredients for compounding
- Thermometers in the refrigerator, freezer, and general pharmacy space
- Air samplers in clean rooms
- Machinery used to compound medications

Always follow the manufacturer's instructions when calibrating equipment.

Infection Control

Infection control is the practice of instituting policies within a healthcare facility to prevent transmission of **communicable diseases**. The policies help prevent employee to employee transmission, employee to patient transmission, patient to employee transmission, and patient to patient transmission. Most facilities have a specific department entirely devoted to developing and monitoring **quality control** techniques and policies within the system to determine their efficacy. Healthcare-related infection is a serious problem in hospitals, especially since hospital-acquired infections may be more dangerous than infections acquired elsewhere. Healthcare-acquired infections are also known as **nosocomial infections**.

Hospital Infection Control Officer

An infection control officer in a hospital or other healthcare setting is typically a doctor, RN, or epidemiologist who has specialized in the prevention of disease transmission. The goal of this position is to prevent transmission of communicable disease in the hospital. The officer achieves this goal by creating policies and practices throughout the hospital, training staff in the policies, and monitoring staff for compliance. Infection control officers may work independently or as part of a larger **infection control team**. Large hospitals often have large infection control teams and may have teams specifically dedicated to preventing infection in each department, including pharmacy.

Infection Control Procedures

Some of the most common infection control **procedures** and **policies** likely to be found in a hospital or other healthcare system include:

- Teaching of proper hand washing technique and provision of multiple stations to accommodate and encourage frequent hand washing
- Aseptic medication preparation and administration
- Providing personal protective equipment, including masks, gloves, gowns, and more
- Ensuring proper sterilization of equipment through the use of alcohol and other disinfectants or autoclaves
- Tracking vaccination records of employees
- Making seasonal vaccinations easily accessible
- Requiring periodic testing for communicable diseases like tuberculosis
- Writing and posting a plan for bloodborne pathogen exposure
- Policies for management of infectious waste
- Investigating any outbreaks that may occur
- Providing prophylactic treatment in case of an accidental exposure

Sharps

In the medical setting, any device that has the potential to break the skin and is a risk for injury and bloodborne pathogen transmission is known as a **sharp**. In most situations, sharps refer to needles used for injections, but can also refer to razor blades, broken glass, scalpels, and other such devices. Sharps must be disposed of according to **proper procedures** to prevent injury, particularly to employees who must handle garbage. Personal protective equipment may not be enough to prevent injuries due to sharps because needles and other sharps can typically cut through medical gloves. Careful handling and proper disposal are the only ways to prevent injuries due to sharps.

Recapping Needles

In most situations, needles should **not** be recapped. This practice often leads to injuries, including sticks and accidental injection of medication. If a situation should arise when a needle must be recapped, never recap a needle by holding the needle in one hand and the cap in the other. Either use tongs to hold the cap, or lay the cap on a flat surface and slide the needle into it. Always properly **dispose** of needles in an appropriate sharps disposal container. It is very important to report any needle stick or injury immediately to both your supervisor and infection control officer.

Disposal of Sharps

Sharps should always be **disposed** of in an approved manner. Special **containers** designed to hold used sharps are available for purchase through pharmacies and medical supply stores and are available in different sizes. These containers can then be dropped off at a designated location for disposal, including hospitals, doctors' offices, pharmacies, and others. Products that destroy needles and make them safe for disposal are also available. Examples include devices that melt or sever the needle, rendering it harmless. Each state has laws regarding the safe disposal of sharps, so it is important to research local laws to be sure that you are following them.

Good Customer Service

Patients who are coming to a pharmacy for services are ill, in pain, or having some other problem or concern. Providing **good customer service** and helping them to feel more at ease goes a long way toward improving the situation for them. Although patients may seem aggravated or short-tempered, it is essential that the person who is assisting them remember that a customer's frustration or anger is generally not directed at them. Additionally, other factors that can make pharmacy experiences frustrating are long lines and waits, issues with insurance companies, and the occasional need to clarify a prescription with the prescriber, which may prolong their wait. Remaining calm and handling situations that arise proactively will go a long way toward improving the overall pharmacy experience for the customer.

Ensuring Good Customer Service

Some ways to ensure good customer service in a pharmacy:

- Offer extra assistance to people who appear to be sick or in pain. Offer a drink or a place to sit while they wait.
- Never argue with customers. Always remain calm and polite. If a customer should become abusive, notify a pharmacist or other supervisor for assistance.
- Avoid using slang terms when assisting elderly patients. Many may not understand what you mean or may be offended.
- Offer to assist anyone who looks like he or she needs help.
- Keep your face and manner neutral, regardless of the medication being dispensed or picked up. Never allow personal feelings or judgment to show.
- Give the patient your full attention. Do not type or answer the phone when you are assisting a customer.
- If you do not know the answer to a question, find someone who does.

Better Customer Service to Senior Citizens

In a pharmacy, many of the patients will be **senior citizens**. Some ways a pharmacy technician can provide better customer service to senior citizens are:

- Speak slowly and enunciate, as they may be hard of hearing.
- Use easy to understand language, and avoid slang and medical jargon.
- Provide a place for them to sit while waiting.
- Listen carefully when they are speaking.
- Many senior citizens may no longer drive and may be waiting for a ride. Try to get their prescription ready quickly.
- Check profiles carefully for polypharmacy and potential interactions. Point these out to the pharmacist for additional counseling opportunities.

Pharmacy Chain of Command

In a typical retail pharmacy setting, especially in a chain store, the **chain of command** works as follows:

1. Pharmacy clerk or assistant
2. Pharmacy technician (uncertified)
3. Pharmacy technician (certified)
4. Lead technician
5. Pharmacy intern
6. Pharmacist

7. Pharmacy supervisor
8. District pharmacy supervisor
9. Regional pharmacy supervisor

When a concern arises, it is important to work up the chain of command. Try to solve problems **locally** (within the location) first. If the problem cannot be solved or if the problem is with the person directly higher in the chain of command, then you may need to work up the chain. Not all steps in the chain will necessarily be present.

Hospital Pharmacy Chain of Command

In a typical hospital pharmacy setting, **chain of command** can sometimes be difficult to assess, particularly if the pharmacy has multiple locations or satellites. A technician working in an oncology satellite may have a different supervisor than a technician working in the main filling location. Generally, the chain of command follows this sort of structure:

1. Pharmacy clerk or assistant
2. Pharmacy technician
3. Certified pharmacy technician
4. Lead technician (may be more than one)
5. Pharmacy intern
6. Pharmacist
7. Pharmacy supervisor (may be more than one)
8. Director of pharmacy staff

It is important to learn the chain of command for your individual organization and any variations depending on your location within the organization.

Workflow

Workflow is a way of arranging job duties so that each step in the process flows smoothly into the next, making work more efficient, saving time and energy. Every pharmacy will have their own way of organizing work so that it flows smoothly, and good pharmacies will constantly be looking for ways to update and improve their workflow. Ideally, every step will be completed and flow naturally to the next step in the process, allowing that step to start immediately. Learning the pharmacy's workflow and your own place within it is the first step to performing your duties as required and keeping work from **bottlenecking** or backing up.

Scheduling

The supervising pharmacist may do the **scheduling** or it may be delegated to a technician or other staff member. Many important considerations must be taken into account when scheduling staff in the pharmacy. The most important principle of scheduling is making sure that there are enough personnel available to **complete the work** promptly and efficiently while staying within **budget restraints**. This means that it is important for staff to show up for their scheduled shifts on time and stay through the entire shift. Failing to show up for a shift puts an unnecessary burden on other staff members and can significantly impede workflow.

Cross Training

In most pharmacies, pharmacy technicians are required to perform a number of functions. While retail pharmacies usually expect pharmacy technicians to perform all necessary duties, technicians in a hospital setting are frequently trained in one area until they have mastered those duties so that jobs are performed as efficiently as possible. However, it is beneficial to the pharmacy to have technicians trained to work in many areas of the pharmacy. This provides more options for scheduling and increased flexibility within the pharmacy. Requesting to be **cross-trained** in other areas of the pharmacy will increase your value as an employee and allow you to build your knowledge and experience.

Multitasking

Multitasking is the ability to perform more than one duty at the same time, for example, entering a prescription while answering a customer's question on the phone, or greeting a customer while ringing out another customer. While multitasking offers the benefit of getting more work done, it can also have some serious drawbacks. When two tasks that demand **accuracy** are performed simultaneously, each task is likely to suffer. You should always give your **full attention** to tasks such as counting medication, compounding medications, IV admixture, or order entry. Having to redo work done incorrectly wastes time. Additionally, performing another task while attending to a customer can cause the customer to feel like they are not important or worth your full attention, which can lead to lost business. One of the few exceptions to this is taking a moment to acknowledge customers that have just arrived. Break what you are doing, tell the customer you will be with them shortly, and then return to your project, double-checking your accuracy due to the interruption.

First Aid Kit

First aid kits are a necessary item that must always be kept in the pharmacy. According to the Red Cross, the items that should be in every first aid kit include:

- Absorbent compresses
- Adhesive bandages
- Adhesive cloth tape
- Antibiotic ointment
- Antiseptic wipes
- Aspirin
- Hydrocortisone ointment
- Instant cold compresses
- Instruction booklet
- Non-latex gloves
- Roller bandages
- Sterile gauze pads
- Thermometer
- Triangular bandages
- Tweezers

First aid kits are available for purchase as a unit or assembled individually. Check the first aid kit when you check expiration dates on the rest of the **pharmacy inventory**. It may be helpful to make a label listing the earliest expiration date in the kit so that it can be replaced as necessary.

Fire Extinguisher

Know the locations of every **fire extinguisher** in the pharmacy. Read the instructions carefully, and understand the use of the extinguisher before an emergency occurs. The instructions for using a fire extinguisher are often identified by the acronym **PASS**:

- **Pull** the pin on top of the extinguisher to unlock it.
- **Aim** the nozzle of the extinguisher at the base of the fire. This will ensure that the fuel is eliminated, preventing the fire from spreading.
- **Squeeze** the lever in a slow and controlled motion.
- **Sweep** from side to side. Start from a safe distance, and move in closer as the fire diminishes.

Accidental Finger Stick

When working with needles, **finger sticks** are a real possibility. If a finger stick occurs while preparing medications, the possibility of injecting yourself with the medication exists. In the case of some medications, this could be very dangerous. If a finger stick occurs, notify your supervisor immediately, and follow these steps:

- Encourage bleeding to help flush out the injected medication.
- Wash the area with soap and water.
- Follow your organization's policies for medical treatment. You may also require a tetanus shot.

If you are accidentally stuck with a needle used on a patient, you will follow these same steps, but the **HIV status** of the person who was previously stuck with the needle will need to be determined. Notify your infection control supervisor immediately. You will likely need to begin **post-exposure prophylaxis**.

Post-Exposure Prophylaxis

Post-exposure prophylaxis, often abbreviated as **PEP**, is treatment and medication provided to someone following potential exposure to HIV, with the goal being to reduce the possibility of developing HIV. Ideally, treatment should begin within the hour following exposure. Protocol typically includes a regimen of **anti-retroviral medications** and follow-up testing and treatment. Although the risk of transmission through a needle stick or other sharps contact is less than one percent, **infection control** should be notified immediately so the incident can be documented and treatment can begin promptly. While PEP can help prevent transmission, it is better to practice safe needle handling techniques to prevent needle sticks and other accidental exposure from occurring at all.

Good Personal Hygiene

Personal hygiene is extremely important in all areas of the healthcare field, including pharmacy. **Clothes** should be clean and free from stains, **hair** should be washed and pulled back, **facial hair** should be neatly trimmed (check with the policies of your location as some health care facilities do not allow facial hair), and hands should always be clean. Not only are you representing your organization to customers and patients who may be turned off by a messy appearance, you are handling medications and medical equipment. Dirty hands can contaminate the medication or equipment. Loose hair may fall into medications or brush equipment. Clean clothes prevent transmission of bacteria and are an important infection control measure.

Healthy Pharmacy Technician

If you are sick with a **viral or bacterial infection**, you should not come to work. Not only do you risk getting the rest of your coworkers sick, you could also infect patients, who may have weakened immune systems due to their own health conditions or treatment. This is especially crucial for pharmacy technicians preparing **chemotherapy** or working in **oncology satellites**. A technician can come to work with a mild cold, although it will be necessary to wear a mask and avoid contact with patients with weakened immune systems. Notify a supervisor if you are not feeling well.

Evaluate Employees

Typically, employees are **evaluated** on a six-month or annual basis. Several processes are used to provide evaluations, including:

- **Supervisor evaluations**, in which the supervisor rates the employee in a number of different areas and lists areas in which the employee excels and areas which may need improvement
- **Peer evaluations**, in which the coworkers of the employee are asked to rate him or her
- **Self-evaluations**, in which employees are asked to rate themselves, including both their strong points and areas in which they may need improvement

Observational data may be used as well as **concrete, numerical data**, depending on the type of position. Pharmacy technician **ratings** typically include accuracy, efficiency, knowledge, and customer service skills.

Self-Evaluations vs. Peer Evaluations

Peer evaluations are helpful when performing employee evaluations because coworkers can often identify strengths and weaknesses that might not be as easily apparent to a supervisor. **Self-evaluations** are often considered the most challenging type of evaluations. Employees are asked to describe their own strengths as well as to identify areas that need improvement. While it may be tempting to list only strengths, it is better to list areas in which you do feel weak, as this is a good opportunity to communicate with your employer, show your desire for improvement, and ask for assistance. Employers appreciate employees who take initiative for their own improvement and training.

Medication Order Entry and Fill Process

Ways a Pharmacy Receives a Valid Prescription

A prescription may be:

- Brought in by a patient or a patient's representative
- Phoned in by a doctor or a doctor's representative
- Faxed
- Transmitted electronically
- Transferred between pharmacies, via pharmacist-to-pharmacist communication
- Requested directly by the patient or patient's representative, via the pharmacy's refill request system or over the phone

Prescriptions may also be accepted through the process of clarifying unclear information. **Limitations** include a) a CII medication may not be received via fax or electronic transfer (although this is allowed in certain situations) and b) a pharmacist must confirm the correctness of a prescription received via phone or electronically.

Processing a Patient's Prescription

When a prescription arrives at the pharmacy, it is **processed** as follows:

- The prescription and all information it contains is entered into the patient's profile.
- The appropriate product is selected for filling the prescriptions.
- The product required to fill the prescriptions is obtained from stock.
- The correct quantity is calculated and dispensed.
- The finished product is appropriately packaged.
- The prescription label and any necessary auxiliary labels are affixed to the container.
- Any necessary patient information materials are collected and assembled.
- The prescription is checked for accuracy (for example, by checking the NDC number).
- Medication and prescription are prepared for final check.

All information is checked by a tech or a pharmacist according to the relevant law.

Medication Calculation

To **calculate** the quantity of a medication correctly, the days' supply and the dosing directions are required. If both of these are available, multiply the **days' supply** by the **number of doses required per day**. For example, if the prescription indicates the patient is to take the medication three times daily for seven days, the amount dispensed would be 21.

To calculate the days' supply of a medication, the number of doses to be dispensed and the dosing directions are required. If both of these are available, divide the **total number of doses** to be dispensed by the **number of doses per day**. For example, if the total number of doses to be dispensed is 28, and the patient is taking two doses per day, the days' supply would be 14.

Prescription Label Information

The following information is required to be listed on the **prescription label**:

- Dispensing pharmacy's name, address, and telephone number
- Directions for use

- Dispensing pharmacist's name or initials
- The prescription serial number
- The medication's name
- The date of the fill or refill
- The medication's strength
- Prescriber's name
- Quantity of medication dispensed
- Patient's name

Most pharmacies use **software** that automatically generates prescription labels that contain all of this information. However, in the case of a software or power failure, the information should be **handwritten** onto the label. Technicians should be familiar with the information that must be included.

Auxiliary Label

The auxiliary label is a label that contains extra information about the medication not given on the prescription label, including additional warnings and qualifications. Common auxiliary labels provide information about **storage**, **unusual routes of administration**, food or water requirements, and **warnings about potentially dangerous side effects**. It is generally agreed that no more than **three** auxiliary labels should be placed on the bottle, although the size of the bottle may also limit the number of labels. Auxiliary labels must be placed in such a way that they do not obscure any of the required information on the prescription labels. Some of the most common auxiliary labels include:

- Do not crush
- Do not drink alcoholic beverages while taking this medication
- May cause drowsiness
- Store in refrigerator
- Take with food
- Medication should be taken with water
- For the nose
- For the ears

Informational Products

A number of **informational products** and brochures may be required to accompany the prescription when given to the patient. Some medications are legally required to have "**black box warning**" information sheets given to patients to explain potentially dangerous side effects. **HIPAA literature** should also accompany each prescription. Printed information about the medication being dispensed is also required to for each new prescription given to the patient and should include information about potential side effects and specific dosing directions. These patient handouts are not intended to replace counseling by the pharmacist.

Tech Check Tech

In some scenarios, pharmacy technicians are allowed to **check** another technician's work. Laws allowing this vary from state to state. In many cases, the technicians allowed to check other technicians have received extra training on the process. In other cases, technicians are checking fills prior to a final check by a pharmacist. Some refill centers also allow the practice, as a pharmacist has already checked the original prescription. "**Tech check tech**" programs are not used in community pharmacies, but may be found in hospital pharmacies, long-term care pharmacies, or other institutional settings.

IV Solution Flow Rate Calculation

Flow rate, or drip rate, of IV solutions is calculated in mL/hr. To determine the mL/hr. for any solution, you must know the total **volume** of the bag to be infused (for example, 1000 mL) and the **time** over which it is to be infused (for example, 8 hours). In this example, you would divide the total mL of the bag by the number of hours, for a flow rate of 125 mL/hr. If the time over which the solution is to be infused is less than an hour, you divide the mL to be infused by the number of minutes over which it is to be infused, then multiply by 60. For example, if a 150 mL piggyback is to be infused over 30 minutes, divide 150 by 30 to get 5. Multiply 5 by 60 to get 300. The flow rate is 300 mL/hr.

Distributing Medication

When medications are to be **distributed** to a patient in the community setting, the following steps to be followed:

- Store the medication properly prior to distribution.
- Make sure that all supplemental information is prepared.
- If you do not know the patient, confirm the patient's identity, by either requesting identification or requesting that the patient confirm birthdate or address. Follow your location's procedure.
- If a patient's representative is picking up the medication, it may be necessary to confirm that this person has permission to pick up the patient's prescription. Again, follow your location's procedure.
- Deliver the medication to the patient or patient's representative.
- Provide pharmacist counseling to the patient.
- Record the distribution as legally required.

Reconstituting Powder for Oral Suspension

Many medications come in a **powder form** that requires **reconstitution** to create an **oral suspension**. These medications should be reconstituted at the point of purchase, when the customer is present to pick them up. Reconstituting early can cause the medication to expire too soon. Patients should not reconstitute powders, as incorrect reconstitution could lead to incorrect dosing. Additionally, using tap water to reconstitute could introduce contaminants. Pharmacies have a device for reconstituting medications with **sterile water**. Some use automated systems, while other systems use gravity. Carefully check the amount of water required to reconstitute the medication, as listed on the label of the medication. Either enter this number into the automated system, or fill the reservoir to exactly this amount. Fill the bottle, stopping halfway through to shake and mix (many automated systems allow for a mix halfway through dispensing the water). Thoroughly **shake** the product to ensure that it is completely mixed before dispensing the medication.

Dispensing Investigational Drugs

Some pharmacies, particularly those found in research and university hospitals, dispense **investigational drugs** used for research. Most of the requirements and protocol for dispensing investigational drugs are the same as those for dealing with any prescription drug. The medication requires orders from a doctor, and a valid written prescription. Other requirements that are specific to investigational drugs include:

- Verification of research or study protocol
- Verification of informed consent from the patient
- Record keeping specific to the study medication
- On-site preparation and storage of the product
- Unique disposal requirements for the product

Automatic Stop Order

Automatic stop orders are safety measures prevent medications from being used for too long unnecessarily or beyond a safe amount of time. Many hospitals have automatic stop orders in place for medications such as **short-term narcotics**, **antibiotics**, and medications such as **ketorolac**. Some systems may automatically **discontinue** medication orders if the patient is transferred to a different level of care, such as, in or out of the intensive care unit or to and from surgery. This requires the doctor to reassess and re-write the medication orders. Individual pharmacy policies on automatic stop orders may vary. Check to find out what your pharmacy's protocol is.

Patient Controlled Analgesic

Patient controlled analgesic, often abbreviated to **PCA**, is a medication that is prepared and administered via a programmed **infusion pump**. It allows the patient to administer a prescribed dose of intravenous pain medication when needed for comfort and pain control, while limiting the amount that can be administered to prevent overdose. PCA devices are commonly used following surgery or childbirth, when patients are alert enough to push the **handheld button**. Only the patient to whom the PCA device is attached is allowed to push the button to dispense the medication. Family members, friends, and other visitors may not dispense the medication, even if they think they are helping the patient. If the patient is not alert enough to dispense the medication, then that patient is not a good candidate for a PCA.

Tinted Prescription Bottles

Inside the pharmacy, medication storage bottles are usually **opaque**. Medications are dispensed in bottles that are either opaque or **tinted**. This is because the chemicals in many medications are light sensitive. Excessive exposure to light will cause the medication to **degrade**, affecting its efficacy and longevity. This is called a **photochemical reaction**. While **amber** is probably the most popular prescription bottle color, other colors that are commonly used include **dark brown**, **dark green**, and **red**. If patients wish to use a Mediset or other system to keep track of their medication, one with a tint should be used to protect the integrity of the medication, or it should be kept in a dark cupboard.

Prepackaged Medication

Many pharmacies, especially hospital or clinic pharmacies, purchase medication in bulk containers then **prepack** it into bottles in commonly used dosages for quick dispensing. This process saves the pharmacy money because they can buy the product in bulk. It also saves time because common doses do not have to be counted out repeatedly. The prepacking is checked by a pharmacist, so when it is time to dispense, the pharmacist only has to make sure that the pre-packed medication is the correct dose and quantity prescribed for the patient. Common medications for prepacking include **antibiotics** and **NSAIDs**.

Robotics

Robotics and **automated dispensing systems** are being used more in high volume pharmacies to improve accuracy, reduce manual labor, cut inventory, and reduce the need for checking. Some types of robotics currently being used include the **Robot-Rx** from McKesson and the **Compact Robotic System** (or CRS) from ScriptPro. The goal of using robotics in pharmacy is to free pharmacists and technicians from menial tasks so that they are available to practice more hands-on patient care. Large **central fill locations** that dispense thousands of scripts daily are more likely to have robotic dispensers.

The Baker Cell

The Baker Cell is a device made by McKesson Automation. When a prescription is entered into the interface, the information is transmitted so that the device will dispense the allotted number of pills. The purpose of the system is to speed up the dispensing of medication and save time. A Baker Cell can count up to 600 pills per minute. The use of the cell allows the pharmacy to increase the number of orders dispensed in the pharmacy and frees up the staff for other activities. The system is modifiable and is customizable to fit nearly any pharmacy setup.

Automated TPN Compounding Equipment

Total parental nutrition compounding often takes place in the pharmacy. Because so many components are used in the preparation of TPNs and each component needs to be perfectly accurate, many pharmacies use **automated TPN equipmen**t to reduce the possibility of errors and increase patient safety. These systems allow for order entry by a pharmacist or a technician into a computer, which then calculates the correct dose for dispensing. The process does require monitoring and setup to ensure a sterile preparation and avoid contamination. Some common automated TPN systems that a technician may encounter include the **Nutramix** by Abbot, the **ExactaMix** by Baxa, and the **AutoComp** by Secure.

Pyxis

Pyxis is a very popular brand of **automated dispensing software** used in hospitals and other medical facilities around the country. The systems are easily customized and may be a single small cabinet or a more complex system complete with refrigeration and automated drawers. Pyxis tracks inventory within its system and creates reports that technicians can use to restock inventory as needed. Pyxis can also be integrated with pharmacy software so that nurses are only able to access medications specifically prescribed for a patient and pharmacists and doctors can track medications given. Pyxis systems are highly **secure**, using password protection and integrating higher security measures such as fingerprint scanning to ensure the safety and security of medications stored within.

Infusion Pump

Infusion pumps are programmable devices that control the rate of different types of infusion. The most common use is for **intravenous** infusion, but **subcutaneous** and **epidural** infusions can also be routed through a pump. Infusion pumps can be programmed to inject intermittent doses of medication or can be used to provide continuous infusion. Infusion pumps can also be programmed to allow for patient controlled analgesia. Infusion pumps come in two basic types: large volume pumps, used to infuse solutions such as total parenteral nutrition, and small volume pumps, which can be used to dose medications like insulin.

Total Parenteral Nutrition Solutions

Most total parenteral solutions follow a specific **formula**. This not only makes it easier for the prescriber, it also makes it easier for the person preparing it, since it is possible to batch orders. TPN solutions are divided into two different categories: **2-in-1 solutions**, which include amino acid and dextrose, and **3-in-1 solutions**, which include amino acid, dextrose, and fat. Other common components of TPN solutions are:

- Fluid, often in the form of water
- Electrolytes, which include sodium, calcium, magnesium, potassium, and phosphate
- Vitamins, including A, B-complex, C, D, and folic acid
- Minerals, such as copper, chromium, manganese, and zinc

Pharmacy Inventory Management

Generic Medication

A generic drug is a medication made by a different manufacturer that matches the brand-name medication in the following areas:

- Active ingredient
- Route of administration
- Dosage form
- Intended use
- Strength Quality and performance characteristics

The generic name of the drug is the **nonproprietary** name of the medication. The Food and Drug Administration oversees generic drugs and the manufacturer must demonstrate that they are identical to their brand name counterpart within an acceptable **bioequivalent range**. A generic drug may be substituted for a brand name drug if the generic name has been written on the prescription. It may also be substituted if the prescriber has marked the prescription "**substitution permitted**" or has failed to mark the prescription "**dispense as written**."

Therapeutic Substitution

A therapeutic substitution is a medication that is different than the one originally prescribed. It is **not** the same as a generic substitution in that the medication may not be the same, or the dosage form, route of administration, or performance characteristics may be different. Therapeutic substitution may be done for a number of reasons. The prescriber is usually consulted although this is not necessary under certain conditions. The most common reasons for therapeutic substitution include:

- The third-party payer does not cover the prescribed medication.
- The prescribed medication is too expensive.
- The prescribed medication is unavailable.
- The prescribed medication is less convenient.

NDC Number

The **National Drug Code number** (NDC number) is a 10-digit number that identifies each unique medication intended for human use. The Drug Listing Act of 1972 established NDC numbers. Each segment of the 10-digit code is used to identify an aspect of the medication:

- The first segment is the **labeler code** and identifies the manufacturer of the medication.
- The second segment is the **product code** and identifies the strength and dosage form of the medication.
- The **package code** is the third segment and identifies the quantity and packaging type of the medication.

An NDC number may not be reassigned if a product is discontinued. Because each product is uniquely identified by the NDC code, technicians and pharmacists can use the code to improve **patient safety** by comparing the code on the package to the code on the prescription to be sure that the patient is being given the correct medication.

Dispense as Written

When prescribing a medication, the prescriber has the option to direct the pharmacy to **dispense as written**. When the prescription is to be dispensed as written, the pharmacy is required to fill it with the exact medication prescribed, even if a generic form of the medication is available. This could be for a variety of reasons:

- The patient may prefer the brand name medication.
- The prescriber may prefer the brand name medication.
- The patient may have an allergy to one of the inactive ingredients in the generic.

If the medication is not available in the form for which the prescription is written, the pharmacy is obligated to contact the prescriber for permission before making any changes to the prescription.

Refrigerated Medications Storage

Some medications are required to be **stored under refrigeration** in order to maintain **potency**. Every pharmacy must keep a dedicated refrigerator on site for the storage of pharmaceuticals requiring refrigeration. Other items, including food for consumption, are not to be stored in this refrigerator. The temperature of the refrigerator must be kept between **2 and 8 degrees Celsius** (36- and 46-degrees Fahrenheit). The temperature should be monitored and logged regularly to ensure that medications are kept at the correct temperature. Some common medications that require refrigeration include **biological medications** such as insulin, many vaccinations, and some suppositories.

Unit Dose

Hospital pharmacies and pharmacies that serve long-term care facilities often package medications in **unit doses**. Unit dose medications serve three specific functions:

1. They prevent dosing errors.
2. They prevent drug diversion.
3. They save time during drug distribution.

Unit dose packaging is subject to the same rules that apply to other medication packages. The package must contain the patient's name; pharmacy name, address, and phone number; the name of the medication, strength, and directions for use; expiration date; and the quantity contained in the package. When medications are unit dosed, the expiration date must be calculated based on the date they were packaged and may not exceed **six months**, even if the bulk container indicates a later date (if the bulk package indicates an expiration date of less than six months, the unit-dose package must also reflect this date).

Proper Storage Conditions

Medications that do not require refrigeration or other specific handling conditions should be kept at **room temperature**, which is defined as being **between 68- and 77-degrees Fahrenheit**, with limited excursions. However, the mean temperature should remain no higher than 77 degrees. To maintain this temperature, pharmacies should have working heaters and air conditioners as necessary based on local climate. A log should be kept in the pharmacy to track daily temperature. If spikes occur, the system should be inspected promptly, as medications can degrade when repeated exposure to temperature extremes occurs.

Automated Dispensing System

Many pharmacies employ an **automated dispensing system** to speed up the dispensing process and improve accuracy. These systems typically store a large number of individual tablets. The necessary quantity is chosen **digitally** (or the system may be connected to the pharmacy's internal computer system). The system dispenses the requested quantity into a pill bottle, which is then labeled by the technician and checked by the pharmacist. It is crucial that the automated system be refilled with the **correct medication** and that the **final check** is never skipped. If controlled medications are kept in the automated dispensing system, a **second count** by a technician or pharmacist should be performed.

Lot Numbers and Expiration Dates

Every medication and medical supply in the pharmacy is marked with a lot number and an expiration date. **Expiration dates** ensure that all medications stored in the pharmacy are used while the medication is guaranteed to be effective and can be pulled prior to expiration. **Lot numbers** identify in which manufacturer's lot the medication was produced. When **drug recalls** occur, the medications to be removed are identified by lot number and expiration date. Keeping medications in the original package will help to identify which medications to remove from the pharmacy and maintain quality control.

Drug Recalls

Occasionally, mistakes occur in the manufacturing or production of medications. Some situations that may require a **recall** include contamination with other products, the incorrect quantity of ingredients, or labeling errors. In this case, the FDA or the drug manufacturer will recall the medications if there is a danger associated with its use. When this occurs, the pharmacy will be notified. The medication should immediately be **pulled** from the shelves and **sequestered** in the pharmacy, clearly marked as a **recalled product**. Further directions from the manufacturer or FDA will follow to instruct the pharmacy as to how the medication should be returned.

Pneumatic Tube System

A pneumatic tube system is a series of tubes and carriers in hospitals and clinics that allows messages and products to be delivered quickly throughout the hospital without the need for human messengers. The item to be delivered is placed in a padded **carrier**, which snaps shut. The carrier is then placed in its **cradle**, and the destination is selected. The carrier travels through the tube system until it reaches its destination. Many hospital pharmacies use the pneumatic tube system to deliver **stat medications** or **single doses** to different areas throughout the hospital. This leaves staff free to complete other duties. Orders may also be sent to the pharmacy from the floors via the pneumatic tube system.

Medications that should **not** be sent through the pneumatic tube system include:

- Narcotics
- Medications with fragile packaging
- Very expensive medications
- Medications requiring the signature of the recipient
- Chemotherapy

Prescription Not in Stock

Occasionally patients will bring a prescription to the pharmacy that is either **not carried** by the store or temporarily **out of stock**. Follow your pharmacy's policy for handling that situation, or you may do the following to assist the patient:

- If the medication is not an emergency, order the medication from the distributor for pick-up the next day.
- Contact other branches of your pharmacy to see either if you can borrow the medication or if the patient can fill the prescription there.
- Contact competitors to see if you can borrow the medication or send the patient there to fill the prescription. The important thing is to assist the patient in getting the medication as quickly and efficiently as possible.

Stock Rotation

Stock rotation is the process of always using the product with the earliest expiration date first. As new inventory comes in, the product on the shelf should be lined up in such a way that the product that will **expire first** is at the front of the shelf, ensuring that it will be used up first. This serves two important functions in pharmacy:

1. It simplifies the issue of **checking expiration dates**. If the product that is going to expire first is in the front, it is easier to identify and remove expired product preventing it from being dispensed to a patient.
2. Because product that expires earlier is in the front, it will be used earlier, preventing the product from **expiring on the shelf**, therefore, reducing waste and overall operating costs.

Pharmaceutical Procurement Policies

Pharmaceutical procurement can be a balancing act. Pharmacies must obtain and keep a sufficient quantity of medications to treat patients without **shortages** occurring. At the same time, keeping a **surplus** of medication may result in medications **expiring** before they can be used, costing the pharmacy money, as expired medications must be removed. Time is wasted during this removal process, as well as valuable storage space. Procurement policies may vary from pharmacy to pharmacy depending on the demands of the population being served and available storage space. A trained team, featuring experts in pharmacy, finance, purchase, and quality control often performs pharmacy procurement.

Par Level and Reorder Level

Par level and reorder level refer to levels of stock used to identify both how much product should be ordered to maintain a level necessary to provide service and when to reorder product. **Par level** is the amount that should be maintained on the shelf at all times. Once the product falls below the par level, it should be **reordered**. Par levels can vary greatly depending on the location and size of the pharmacy, the population it serves, and the time that passes between orders. For example, Pharmacy ABC may be a small store serving a relatively young population; their par level of amlodipine may be 300 tablets. At Pharmacy XYZ, a larger store in a part of town with more retirees, the par level may be 3000 tablets.

Receiving Inventory

When the order arrives from the shipper, count the boxes that arrive to confirm that you have received the amount expected. Once the boxes are checked in, open each box, and compare the contents to the **packing slip**. This can be done a number of different ways, depending on the policy of the pharmacy. Some pharmacies will have you check the order **manually**. Larger pharmacies that receive bigger orders may have a **scanning system** set up that allows you to scan the product, which allows the computer to compare it to the invoice and add it to the inventory. Some pharmacy orders come through a home office, and the inventory is updated when the order is received in the computer. In this case, any discrepancies must be manually corrected. Product should be **put away promptly** to prevent mistakes, storage issues, and lost product.

Identify Expired or Unsalable Stock

Most pharmacies have a system or routine built into daily practice to help identify and segregate product that is **expired** or otherwise **unsalable**. One common system is to have technicians assigned to an area of the pharmacy checking on a **monthly basis** for expired or unsalable medication. Another system may assign one technician to check the pharmacy **constantly** for expired medications. All areas of the pharmacy must be checked. Even with systems such as these in place, it is still the responsibility of every staff member to check expiration dates before using any medication to ensure that the medication is safe to use.

Logs

Numerous logs measuring many different variables can be found throughout the pharmacy. Some common ones include:

- Refrigerator and freezer temperatures
- Ambient air temperatures
- Equipment cleaning
- Air cleanliness testing
- Calibration of equipment

These logs are important and should not be neglected. If the pharmacy or refrigerator temperature experiences changes, medication **integrity** could be compromised. It is important to track **routine sanitation jobs** to a) make sure among the staff that they are being done, and b) prove to certification and inspecting organizations that they are being done. Most of this information may need to be provided in case of a **safety audit**, and it is important that records be current and constantly maintained. They should also be easily accessible, and each member of the pharmacy staff should know where to find them.

Pharmacy Billing and Reimbursement

Methods of Payment

A variety of payment methods may be used in a retail pharmacy. The pharmacy technician is responsible for learning how to ring each one up according to the **cash drawer system** used in the individual pharmacy. Payment methods likely to be used are:

- Cash
- Personal check
- Third party check (power of attorney)
- Third party payer (usually done via computer)
- Flexible spending accounts
- Credit and debit cards
- Financial assistance cards issued by the state

While some pharmacies use pharmacy assistants instead of pharmacy technicians to run the cash drawers, everyone in the pharmacy should know how to run the cash drawer and be able to step up to assist if necessary.

Third-Party Payer

A third-party payer is an entity that pays for health care services but is neither the patient nor the medical provider. The most common type of third-party payer is **health insurance**, which can take the form of **private insurance** purchased by the patient or **public health insurance** available through the government. A patient whose prescriptions are paid for through a third party must follow the rules and policies set forth by the third party, which may include limited access to certain medications and treatments. Most third parties are accessible through pharmacy computer systems and are able to provide an approval or denial along with the **amount covered** and the **patient responsibility** at the point of sale. Others will require the patient to pay retail price, and then fill out the appropriate forms and send them in for full reimbursement.

Medicaid and Medicare

Medicaid – Medicaid is the federal program that provides access to health care for **low-income** people or people who meet certain other requirements. Each state manages its own Medicaid program, although costs are shared between each state and the federal government. In addition to medical care and medications, Medicaid also provides dental care and a screening program called Early and Periodic Screening, Diagnostic and Treatment that helps to identify and diagnose children with medical conditions.

Medicare – Medicare is the federal program that provides insurance and health care to people **over age 65** or people who meet other criteria, such as permanent disability, cognitive disability, or certain other conditions. Medicare consists of four different services. These services are:

- **Medicare Part A**: Hospital Insurance
- **Medicare Part B**: Medical Insurance
- **Medicare Part C**: Medicare Advantage Programs
- **Medicare Part D**: Prescription Drug Program

Denied Medication Claim

Medication claims can be **denied** by third-party payers for a number of reasons. When a claim has been denied, patients still have some options. Some of the options available are:

- The prescriber can be contacted to prescribe a different drug.
- The patient may opt to pay for the medication out of pocket (though this is not an option if the claim was denied because the refill is too soon).
- The patient may appeal the claim to the insurance company.
- The patient may request a special authorization for the medication.

Third-Party Payer Rejection

A number of small mistakes may cause a prescription to be **rejected** by the third-party payer. Many of these mistakes can be easily found and corrected by the pharmacy technician. When a prescription is rejected, check for these potential problems:

- The patient's name doesn't match
- The patient's birthday doesn't match
- The patient's gender doesn't match
- The days' supply is incorrect or unusual for the medication
- The prescription has been recently filled at another pharmacy (this may also indicate drug-seeking behavior on the part of the patient)
- The prescription is being refilled too soon
- The days' supply is higher than allowed by the insurance company.

Some of these errors occur at the level of the **insurance company**. For example, birthday and gender errors are not uncommon. If this is the case, it may be necessary to temporarily change the information in the pharmacy database to run the prescription until the insurance company can fix the error on their end.

Prior Authorization

Before paying for a medication, some insurance companies will require a process known as **prior authorization**. This means that the medication is only eligible for coverage if the patient meets a certain predetermined set of **guidelines**. The insurance company must be contacted, and a case must be presented as to why the patient requires this medication and cannot use a **formulary substitution**. The insurance company will then make the decision based on the information provided as to whether they will cover that medication for the patient. Different insurance companies have different rules, including who must make the request for authorization and how it is to be made.

Formulary

A formulary is a list of medications preferred by an organization. A hospital will have a drug formulary, as will an insurance company. Formularies are usually created as a means of **controlling costs** and are designed by doctors and pharmacists within the organization. Hospitals may switch a patient from a **non-formulary medication** to an equivalent **formulary medication** while he or she is an inpatient. An insurance company may require prior authorization or approval before covering a medication that is not on their formulary of preferred medications or may deny it outright. Patients who are covered by an insurance company are provided access to the company's formulary via the company's written materials or website. Patients are responsible for being familiar with the contents of their insurance company's formulary.

Co-Pay

The co-pay is the portion of the payment for which the patient is responsible after the insurance company has paid its share. Co-pays are highly variable depending on the insurance company, the individual prescription plan, and the type of medication. Most insurance companies have a **tiered system**, where preferred medications and generics are a lower price, while non-preferred medications cost more. In most cases, submitting the medication to the insurance company via the online computer system will provide the correct co-pay for the medication. Patients are responsible for knowing the formulary and tiers of their insurance company.

Register Scanned No Co-Pay Prescription

In some cases, a prescription will have **no co-pay**. Most pharmacy systems will still require the prescription to be **scanned** at the register when the patient picks it up. This is done for a few reasons:

- It creates a record in the system of the medication being picked up.
- The prescription must be sold through the system to allow a patient to sign for the prescription.
- It changes the pharmacy's inventory to reflect the medication being sold.
- Procedures vary from store to store, so follow your pharmacy's policy.

No Co-Pay Prescription

When a patient's prescription is submitted to their insurance company, occasionally it may come back with a **zero co-pay**. A patient may have a prescription with no co-pay for a few different reasons:

- Patients who receive prescription assistance through the state often have no co-pay.
- Coupon programs provided by the manufacturer will often result in a zero co-pay.
- Some prescription plans cover certain maintenance medications 100 percent, resulting in a zero co-pay.

If the patient was expecting a zero co-pay, it may be necessary to **contact the insurance company** to find out the company's rules for that medication. If you have time, contacting the insurance company on the patient's behalf is a good way to provide customer service, but ultimately it is the **patient's responsibility** to know his or her insurance plan.

Insurance Card

The information provided on **insurance company cards** varies, but there are a few pieces of information typically available on every card and are crucial to running the prescription. These are:

- The patient's name
- The member ID (including any additional digits such as -00, -01, etc. These numbers identify the patient's relationship to the subscriber)
- The RXPCN
- The BIN
- The group name or number

The information required will vary based on the pharmacy computer system and the insurance company. Some insurance cards contain information about co-pays. The back of the card usually contains information such as the address and phone number of the insurance company, which can be helpful when a problem arises.

Insurance Subscriber and Dependents

The insurance subscriber is the person who owns the insurance policy. If the insurance is through an employer, the subscriber is the **employee** who works for the employer. If the insurance has been purchased individually, the subscriber is the person who **purchased** the policy and is responsible for making the payments. **Dependents** are other people who also receive coverage on the policy. Dependents may include:

- Spouse
- Minor children
- Stepchildren
- Children up to age 26 who don't have access to another health insurance plan

Laws vary depending on the state. Check current coverage laws to find out who is allowable as a dependent on health insurance.

Billing Services Procedure

In some cases, insurance companies will pay for services, but only by **reimbursing** the customer. Although patients are primarily responsible for this procedure, pharmacy technicians can assist and provide guidance.

- Contact the insurance company to find out their procedure. Some allow reimbursement requests to be filed online; others will provide paperwork that will need to be filled out.
- Confirm that the services are in fact reimbursable.
- Print out receipts or other required proof of services rendered.
- Locate the address to which the information should be mailed or faxed.

ICD Codes

ICD codes are standardized numerical codes are used to differentiate between different medical conditions. ICD stands for **International Statistical Classification of Diseases and Related Health Problems**. In the pharmacy, ICD codes may be required for billing of some medications to insurance companies. In some cases, insurance companies will only pay for medications prescribed to treat a specific condition. The ICD code is then submitted to the insurance company electronically or as part of a prior authorization request. Doctors sometimes write the ICD code on the prescription, but in many cases, the pharmacy will have to contact the doctor to request the ICD code.

Some samples of ICD codes include:

- 780.30 Seizures NOS
- 733.00 Osteoporosis
- 572.80 Liver disease – hepatic failure

Flexible Spending Account

Many insurance companies offer subscribers the option of a flexible spending plan or **flexible spending account** as one of their health insurance options. This option deducts money from the patient's pre-tax income into an account that can then be used to pay for **healthcare-related expenses** in order to avoid paying **taxes** on that money. The money must be used within the specified amount of time, or it goes away. One of the benefits of a flexible spending account is that it can be used to pay for over-the-counter products and co-pays. Flexible spending account rules vary, and it is the patient's responsibility to know the policies and limitations of his or her flexible spending plan.

Products Purchased with a Flexible Spending Account

Numerous products in the pharmacy can be purchased using a **flexible spending account**, although the rules for doing so vary from state to state and from plan to plan. The patient is responsible for knowing which products can be purchased on his or her plan, although some cards will deny attempts to use them to purchase unauthorized products. Some of the products that may be eligible include:

- Over the counter medications used to treat a number of conditions, with a doctor's prescription
- Diabetes testing supplies, including strips, alcohol wipes, and more
- Syringes for injecting medications
- Bandages and other first-aid necessities
- Other items that would be deductible as medical tax expenses

Pharmacy Information System Usage and Application

Automated Medication-Dispensing Devices

Automated medication-dispensing devices are often used in hospital settings to store medications on the patient care unit so that nurses have convenient access for patients' doses. These systems also serve to ensure **patient and medication safety** and to prevent **drug diversion**. These devices store the medications in a cabinet that is locked and only accessible with a unique **identifier** and **password**. More advanced models are able to use technology like fingerprint scanning to identify authorized users. The system tracks the doses given to patients as well as the users who are accessing the cabinet. Advanced systems send reports to a central unit, which pharmacy staff can access to check the status of any unit in the system and to determine which units need to be stocked. Common manufacturers of these systems include Pyxis, Baxter, and McKesson.

FDA Med Watch Program

The FDA MedWatch Program is an online system that allows for reporting of **adverse events** due to medications and other medical products. Both consumers and healthcare professionals can make reports. In addition to serious adverse effects, other information requested includes problems with product quality, mistakes made in product use, or failures of medications considered therapeutically equivalent. Additionally, subscribers receive safety alerts on medications as they are posted. The aim of this program is to increase the ease of reporting to improve consumer safety and quickly get information about **potential safety issues** out to the public.

PTCB Practice Test

1. Which of the following is the most correct transcription of the prescription directions of "1 tablet QD"?

a. Take one tablet two times daily.
b. Take one tablet four times daily.
c. Take one tablet daily.
d. Take one tablet three times daily.

2. Which of the following is an error-reducing procedure for writing numbers?

a. Place a terminal period after mg (e.g., 50 mg.).
b. Preface numbers less than one with a zero (e.g., 0.5 mg).
c. Add a zero after whole numbers (e.g., 5.0 mg).
d. Do not add a zero before a number less than one (e.g., .5 mg).

3. If a chemotherapy spill occurs inside the hood, what measure should NOT always be taken?

a. Double glove, don gown, and put on eye protection.
b. Turn off blower.
c. Leave blower on.
d. Clean liquid spill with absorbent (e.g., gauze).

4. Which of the following is NOT an example of quality assurance in inventory control?

a. denoting high-alert medications
b. using electronic prescription capabilities
c. using bar-code procedures during prescription filling
d. double-checking work

5. Which of the following describes requirements for the stability of sterile products?

a. USP <797>
b. TJC
c. SDS
d. OSHA

6. What test can monitor the use of enoxaparin?

a. INR
b. aPTT
c. RBC
d. antifactor Xa

7. What must a clinician be concerned about regarding the combination of Proscar and Prozac?

a. drug – drug interaction
b. IV incompatibility
c. schedule IV drugs
d. look-alike, sound-alike drug name pair

8. Which of the following drug combinations is NOT contraindicated?

a. Demerol – Nardil
b. aspirin – Coumadin
c. Zerit – Retrovir
d. Reclast – Actonel

9. What condition does a patient requiring Pancrease likely have?

a. cystic fibrosis
b. asthma
c. renal failure
d. osteoporosis

10. What is the dose of gentamicin 2 mg/kg for a patient weighing 175 lbs?

a. 120 mg
b. 160 mg
c. 180 mg
d. 200 mg

11. A patient is to receive 100 mg/m^2 of docetaxel. What is the appropriate dose for a patient weighing 175 pounds with a body surface area of 1.8m^2?

a. 180 mg
b. 360 mg
c. 4400 mg
d. 8,000 mg

12. In a horizontal flow hood, how far should one work inside the hood?

a. 4 inches
b. 6 inches
c. 10 inches
d. 12 inches

13. Crushed or broken tablets of which prescription medication should NOT be handled by a pharmacy technician who is pregnant?

a. furosemide
b. famotidine
c. finasteride
d. fluoxetine

14. What can direct mixture of calcium gluconate and potassium phosphate solutions for injection cause?

a. lactated Ringer's solution
b. emulsion
c. precipitate
d. suspension

15. Which auxiliary label should NOT be applied to a prescription label on Biaxin oral suspension?

a. Shake well.
b. Refrigerate.
c. Finish the entire course.
d. Take on an empty stomach.

16. Which of the following ingredients of TPN may interact with warfarin?

a. potassium chloride (KCl)
b. multivitamins
c. lipids
d. vitamin K

17. A patient presents you with a prescription for clozapine. What is NOT true regarding clozapine prescriptions?

a. Registration prior to dispensing or prescribing is required.
b. Patients require frequent monitoring of the absolute neutrophil count (ANC) and white blood cell (WBC) count.
c. Clozapine is only available through a distribution system.
d. Clozapine is indicated for severe depression.

18. Which herbal preparation is often used for depression?

a. St. John's wort
b. echinacea
c. saw palmetto
d. valerian

19. Which of the following is NOT an example of a drug and one of its appropriate monitoring parameters?

a. metoprolol – heart rate
b. filgrastim – triglycerides
c. zoledronic acid – creatinine
d. fluorouracil – WBC

20. How should regular insulin be combined with NPH insulin in the same syringe?

a. Add regular insulin to syringe first, then add NPH.
b. Add NPH to syringe first, then add regular insulin.
c. These cannot be combined in the same syringe.
d. It doesn't matter which one is added first.

21. How should used fentanyl patches be discarded?

a. mixing in coffee grounds before disposing
b. returning to the pharmacy
c. flushing in the toilet
d. throwing in regular trash

22. Which of the following is NOT something a patient receiving rifampin should be counseled about?

a. blue-green discoloration of urine
b. permanent discoloration of contact lenses
c. drug–drug interactions
d. decreased effectiveness of birth control pills

23. A patient receives a prescription for oxycodone/acetaminophen 5/325. What is the maximum number of tablets the patient may take daily?

a. 6
b. 8
c. 10
d. 12

24. Where is medication recall information NOT located?

a. fax from manufacturer
b. letter from wholesaler
c. FDA website
d. DEA website

25. When double-checking a computer entry of a drug versus its National Drug Code (NDC) number, which part of the NDC should be compared to the drug entry?

a. digits 1 through 5
b. digits 6 through 9
c. digits 10 through 11
d. all 11 digits

26. Which of the DEA numbers listed below would be a valid number for general medical practitioner Dr. Shannon Brinks?

a. FB2146339
b. SB2146335
c. BS2146333
d. BB2146337

27. Drug ABC is an investigational drug for psoriasis. What is NOT the physician's responsibility regarding drug ABC?

a. Obtain signed consent.
b. Obtain study approval from the IRB.
c. Store drug ABC.
d. Provide pharmacy with a signed consent form.

28. How many milliliters of a 10 mg/mL oral solution should be dispensed for a patient requiring two teaspoonfuls three times daily for seven days?

a. 105 mL
b. 210 mL
c. 315 mL
d. 630 mL

29. A patient requires 20 mEq/L of potassium phosphate. How many milliliters of a 4.4 mEq/mL concentrated solution should be added to a bag containing 500 mL?

a. 1 mL
b. 2.3 mL
c. 4.5 mL
d. 23 mL

30. Labels on repackaged medication (e.g., unit dose) must contain all EXCEPT which of the following?

a. manufacturer lot number
b. expiration date
c. patient's name
d. drug generic name

31. All prescription labels must contain which of the following?

a. physician telephone number
b. date prescription written
c. name of drug distributor
d. name of drug manufacturer

32. You are filling a prescription for Toprol XL to be taken once daily for one year. The insurance company requires that a three-month supply be filled. How many refills will the patient have?

a. 1
b. 3
c. 4
d. 11

33. Which of the following drugs contains acetaminophen?

a. Roxicet
b. Vicoprofen
c. Fiorinal
d. Darvon

34. Which of the following forms is used for the transfer of schedule II medications between institutions?

a. DEA Form 222
b. DEA Form 41
c. DEA Form 106
d. DEA Form 224

35. Which of the following is the correct combination of a drug and its antidote?

a. aspirin – N-acetylcysteine
b. potassium chloride – vitamin K
c. methotrexate – dexrazoxane
d. midazolam – flumazenil

36. What is an advantage of diphenhydramine oral solution versus diphenhydramine capsules?

a. no taste
b. faster onset of action
c. easier to transport
d. more convenient

37. Which is of the following NOT something all pharmacies must have?

a. class B balance
b. class A balance
c. mortar and pestle
d. pharmacy weights

38. What is a responsibility specific to an institutional pharmacy technician?

a. Maintain inventory.
b. Prepackage bulk medications.
c. Inspect nursing unit.
d. Assist the pharmacist.

39. If requested, filed prescriptions must be retrievable within how many hours?

a. 24 hours
b. 36 hours
c. 48 hours
d. 72 hours

40. What percentage of dextrose and sodium chloride are in a liter of D5NS?

a. dextrose 5%, sodium chloride 0.9%
b. dextrose 5%, sodium chloride 0.45%
c. dextrose 5%, sodium chloride 0.225%
d. dextrose 5%, no sodium chloride

41. When making IVs, which part of the syringe must never be touched?

a. barrel
b. barrel flange
c. plunger
d. shaft

42. What is the brand name for insulin glargine?

a. Lantus
b. NovoLog
c. Apidra
d. Levemir

43. Which of the following is a C-II?

a. Dolophine
b. Restoril
c. Strattera
d. Suboxone

44. Which of the following agents is an antibacterial?

a. fluconazole
b. nystatin
c. doxycycline
d. acyclovir

45. What is Patanol indicated for?

a. high blood pressure
b. conjunctivitis
c. eye allergies
d. skin allergies

46. Which of the following choices describes a "misbranded" drug?

a. contains unsafe additives
b. differs in strength from what is represented
c. label does not contain directions for use
d. was prepared in unsanitary conditions

47. Which of the following is true about the filling of schedule II drugs?

a. A partial filling is allowed if the remaining quantity is available within 48 hours.
b. All prescriptions must be handwritten.
c. An emergency filling is not allowable.
d. Faxed prescriptions may be acceptable from long-term care facilities.

48. Of the following NEW orders sent to your pharmacy, which should be filled "stat"?

a. TPN
b. Cardura XL
c. amikacin
d. Lotrimin

49. Which of the following drugs may be delivered via the pneumatic tube system?

a. magnesium citrate
b. gemcitabine
c. pegfilgrastim
d. abciximab

50. You need to repackage 30 pills from a manufacturer bottle with an expiration date of 3/11. What would be the appropriate expiration date for the repackaged product if the current date is 3/31/10?

a. 9/10
b. 7/10
c. 6/10
d. 12/10

51. What is the generic name of Seroquel?

a. bupropion
b. olanzapine
c. quetiapine
d. venlafaxine

52. What is the brand name of duloxetine?

a. Abilify
b. Cymbalta
c. Lexapro
d. Zyprexa

53. Which type of laminar flow hood exhausts all air to the outside atmosphere after it passes through a HEPA filter?

a. type A
b. type B1
c. type B2
d. type B3

54. Which of the following needles has the smallest bore?

a. 16 G
b. 18 G
c. 19 G
d. 21 G

55. Which of the following is true about a drug involved in a FDA class II recall?

a. may cause serious, permanent adverse effects
b. may cause adverse effects that are temporary
c. may not cause adverse effects
d. was contaminated

56. Which types of solutions may contain alcohol?

a. collodion, tincture, syrup
b. tincture, syrup, spirits
c. aromatic waters, liniments, tincture
d. elixir, spirits, tincture

57. What type of dispersion is Silvadene?

a. cream
b. gel
c. ointment
d. paste

58. What condition is quinine approved for?

a. cardiac arrhythmias
b. leg cramps
c. malaria
d. B and C

59. What drug class does Lioresal belong to?

a. antidiabetic
b. diuretic
c. antipsychotic
d. antispasmodic

60. How many pints are in one gallon?

a. 4
b. 6
c. 8
d. 10

61. Convert 1.33 milligrams to micrograms.

a. 13.3 mcg
b. 133 mcg
c. 1330 mcg
d. 13,300 mcg

62. Interpret this set of Roman numerals: MCLXXIV.

a. 664
b. 1164
c. 1174
d. 1574

63. How many tablespoons are in two cups?

a. 4
b. 8
c. 16
d. 32

64. How many micrograms are in one grain?

a. 6.5
b. 650
c. 6500
d. 65,000

65. What is a hermetic container?

a. tamper resistant
b. impermeable to light
c. heat resistant
d. impermeable to air

66. Which of the following drugs is an oral antineoplastic agent for non-small-cell lung cancer?

a. erlotinib
b. nelarabine
c. vorinostat
d. sorafenib

67. Which corticosteroid is NOT more potent than prednisone?

a. methylprednisolone
b. dexamethasone
c. hydrocortisone
d. prednisolone

68. Which affective disorder is characterized by apprehension and worry?

a. ADHD
b. depression
c. psychosis
d. anxiety

69. Which antiretroviral for human immunodeficiency virus may cause fat redistribution (lipodystrophy)?

a. nelfinavir
b. lamivudine
c. efavirenz
d. enfuvirtide

70. Which of the following references would be a source of information for a drug from Canada?

a. Goodman and Gilman's
b. Remington's
c. Trissel's
d. Martindale's

71. Which of the following is true about Medicare or Medicaid?

a. Medicaid is state-funded health insurance for people ages 65 and older and others with certain disease states.
b. Medicare is state-funded health insurance for people ages 65 and older and others with certain disease states.
c. Medicaid is state-administered health insurance for people and families of low income.
d. Medicare is state-administered health insurance for people and families of low income.

72. Which of the following is true about isotretinoin prescriptions?

a. Only a 30-day supply is allowed.
b. All female patients must have a bimonthly pregnancy test.
c. Isotretinoin is indicated for all types of acne.
d. A CBC count must be obtained monthly for anemia.

73. How many milligrams of hydrocortisone should be used in compounding this prescription?

Rx: Hydrocortisone 0.5%
Hydrophilic ointment ad 10 g

a. 0.5 mg
b. 5 mg
c. 50 mg
d. 500 mg

74. How many 300 mcg tablets of colchicine may be prepared from 3 gm of colchicine?

a. 100
b. 1000
c. 10,000
d. 1000,000

75. What is NOT true regarding the transfer of a prescription for a controlled substance?

a. "VOID" must be written on the face of the original prescription.
b. The original and transferred prescriptions must be archived for one year.
c. The date of issuance of the original prescription must be written on the transferred prescription.
d. C-IIs cannot be transferred.

76. Which dosage form of potassium chloride (KCl) would provide the most accurate delivery of drug to a one-year-old patient?

a. K-Dur
b. K-Lor
c. KCl IV piggyback
d. KCl oral solution

77. Drug A regularly costs $114.00. A drug distributor is offering a discount of 5%. What is the purchase price of drug A?

a. $57.00
b. $108.30
c. $113.43
d. $119.70

78. How many times must inventory be turned over for a business to have what is considered a good rate for financial well-being?

a. 6
b. 10
c. 12
d. 15

79. What is true about controlled substances?

a. An institutional DEA number is not required for return of a controlled substance.
b. DEA Form 222 must be completed prior to destruction of the controlled substance.
c. DEA Form 41 must be completed on the day of destruction.
d. DEA Form 41 copy must be submitted to the DEA prior to destruction of controlled substances.

80. What is NOT true about a group purchasing organization?

a. negotiates with drug manufacturers for discounted drugs
b. purchases discounted drugs for hospitals
c. develops contracts with drug companies
d. assists hospitals, home-health agencies, and nursing homes

81. Who develops the formulary in a hospital?

a. IV room
b. director of the pharmacy
c. TJC
d. P&T committee

82. A hospital P&T committee decides that drug A can be used instead of drug B. What is this process called?

a. therapeutic substitution
b. therapeutic bioavailability
c. therapeutic equivalency
d. therapeutic equality

83. Which of the following is true about personal protective equipment for IV compounding?

a. Jewelry is allowed if latex gloves are worn.
b. Use of makeup is allowed if a mask or face shield is worn.
c. Hands do not need to be washed if latex gloves are worn.
d. Compounding gowns are particulate free.

84. Which of the following is true about the legal and regulatory requirements of medications?

a. The FDA enforces the Controlled Substances Act.
b. The DEA ensures that pharmacy technician requirements are met.
c. The Joint Commission can issue drug recalls.
d. The USP makes requirements for drug labeling.

85. What do the suffixes A-D, XL, and AF mean after the drug names of Imodium A-D, Procardia XL, and Diprolene AF?

a. as directed, extended release, atrial fibrillation
b. as directed, extended release, antifungal
c. antidiarrheal, extended release, antifungal
d. antidiarrheal, extended release, augmented formula

86. What is NOT true about Radioactive Yellow III materials?

a. Radioactive Yellow III contains the lowest concentration of radiation.
b. Radioactive Yellow III requires a metal shipping container for transportation.
c. A special placard must be placed on any vehicle transporting Radioactive Yellow III materials.
d. Shipment is regulated by the U.S. DOT.

87. Which of the following is correct about a HEPA filter?

a. HEPA stands for high-efficiency pharmaceutical appliance.
b. Particles greater than three milligrams are prevented from entering the sterile environment.
c. Cleaning agents can be sprayed on the HEPA filter.
d. The hood should be certified any time the HEPA filter becomes wet.

88. Water is

a. hypertonic
b. osmotic
c. hypotonic
d. isotonic

89. Which of the following is true about compounding equipment?

a. Stainless steel spatulas are used for corrosive ingredients.
b. Digital balances are sensitive to 0.001 mg.
c. Glass mortars and pestles are used for mixing liquid and semisolid ingredients.
d. A volume delivered by a "TD" graduate is inaccurate.

90. Which of the following is true about OBRA 90?

a. requires that all pharmacists perform an MAR
b. requires that pharmacies protect private patient information
c. requires that pharmacies maintain patient profiles
d. requires that patients with disabilities are not discriminated against

Answer Key and Explanations

1. C: According to the Institute for Safe Medication Practices (ISMP), the abbreviation "QD" should never be used in communicating information to other health professionals. Abbreviations should be avoided in all prescription writing and medical communication. Abbreviations have led to many serious medication errors. QD has been mistaken for QID, and fourfold dosing errors have occurred as a result. In addition, numerals should be spelled out.

2. B: Many errors have occurred due to the misreading of prescriptions. A terminal period should not be used after dosing increments, such as mg or mL, due to the possible misinterpretation of the period as the number 1. Trailing zeros should not be added after whole numbers due to the risk of a tenfold overdose if the period is poorly written or hard to see. A zero should be added before a whole number because if the period is not seen, a tenfold overdose may occur (e.g., 5 mg given instead of 0.5 mg).

3. B: In case of a chemotherapy spill inside a hood, several measures should be taken to prevent worker and workplace exposure. The worker cleaning up the spill should don additional protective wear, such as double gloves, eyewear, and a gown. If a liquid is spilled, absorbent gauze or a gauze pillow (from the spill kit) should be placed gently on the spill to avoid splashing. Powder or solid spills should be cleaned using water-soaked gauze. All items used to clean up the spill should be disposed of in yellow chemotherapy bags. The blower should be left on unless the HEPA filter has been contaminated.

4. D: Quality assurance helps guarantee patient safety. Mechanisms to assure patient safety include storing dangerous and high-alert medications separately from regular stock, bar coding all procedures associated with prescription filling, and implementation of computerized physician order entry to minimize poor legibility. All involved with medication filling should triple check their work.

5. A: United States Pharmacopeia (USP) Chapter 797 is a set of sterile compounding standards created in order to reduce the risk of patient infection and to protect employees. Use of USP <797> is required for any institution in which sterile compounding occurs. The Joint Commission (TJC) is an agency that accredits health-care institutions based on patient care and safety standards. Safety Data Sheets (SDSs), provided by product sellers, detail chemical products, potential dangers associated with these chemicals, and measures to be taken in case of exposure. The Occupational Safety and Health Administration (OSHA) is an agency that ensures a safe and healthy workplace.

6. D: The low-molecular-weight heparins (LMWHs), including enoxaparin, generally do not require laboratory monitoring. The international normalized ratio (INR) is used for warfarin monitoring, and the activated partial thromboplastin time (aPTT) is used for heparin monitoring. The red blood cell (RBC) count is a measure of red blood cells, and a low value denotes the presence of anemia (bleeding). If laboratory monitoring of LMWHs is desired (e.g., for patients who are obese or have renal insufficiency), it is usually via antifactor Xa.

7. D: "Proscar and Prozac" are an example of a look-alike, sound-alike (LASA) drug name pair. Such drugs have a risk of being mistaken for each other due to similarities in spelling and/or sound. LASA drugs should not be stored next to each other, and other precautions should be taken to minimize error. Proscar and Prozac are not controlled substances, are oral agents (not administered IV), and do not interact with each other.

8. B: Demerol should never be given with monoamine oxidase inhibitors (MAOIs), such as Nardil, due to the risk of hypertensive crisis and death. Zerit and Retrovir are both nucleoside reverse transcriptase inhibitors used for the treatment of human immunodeficiency virus (HIV). This combination should be avoided due to possible antagonism, rendering treatment ineffective. Reclast and Actonel are both bisphosphonates used for osteoporosis. Reclast is an IV product taken once yearly, and Actonel is an oral product taken once weekly. These agents should not be coadministered due to the risk of toxicity. Aspirin and Coumadin are generally not coadministered together due to the risk of bleeding. However, some patients will require this combination due to their clinical condition. Patients taking both medications should be counseled about signs and symptoms of bleeding.

9. A: Pancrease is a mixture of enzymes normally produced in the pancreas. Cystic fibrosis is a condition in which the body does not supply enough of its own pancreatic enzymes. This does not occur with asthma, renal failure, or osteoporosis.

10. B: First, one must convert pounds to kilograms. Divide 175 lbs by 2.2 kg/lbs to obtain 79.5 kg. Multiply by 2 mg/kg for an answer of 160 mg.

11. A: Body surface area (BSA) is a measurement of the surface of the body using height and weight and is often used for dosing of certain medications, such as chemotherapy. In this instance, the answer is 1.8 m2 × 100 mg/m2 for 180 mg. Weight is unneeded, as it had already been incorporated into the patient's BSA.

12. B: One should work at least six inches inside the hood to ensure adequate sterile compounding and airflow. One should also position hands during compounding in an effort to avoid blocking airflow.

13. C: Women who are pregnant and handling medications should consider taking precautions against drug exposure, such as wearing gloves or a mask. Broken or crushed finasteride should not be handled by a pregnant female due to the risk for fetal harm. Furosemide, famotidine, and fluoxetine do not carry the same precautions regarding handling.

14. C: An emulsion is the mixture of one liquid dispersed with another with the aid of a dispersing agent. An example is fat emulsion used for total parenteral nutrition (TPN). Lactated Ringer's solution is used intravenously or for irrigation and contains sodium, potassium, and calcium salts. A suspension is generally a solid mixed in another vehicle such as glycerin or water (for example, oral azithromycin suspension). The combination of calcium gluconate and potassium phosphate can result in a precipitate, which is a potentially dangerous formation of solid crystals. Caution should be exercised when dosing and admixing these agents for use in IV preparations, such as for TPN.

15. B: Biaxin oral suspension should be shaken well prior to use, may be taken with or without food, and the entire course should be finished. Biaxin oral suspension should not be refrigerated.

16. D: Errors have occurred in which patients receiving warfarin have inadvertently received vitamin K. Vitamin K is often added to TPN once weekly, and this may be missed in patients receiving warfarin during the medication profile review. Vitamin K antagonizes the warfarin anticoagulant activity, rendering it ineffective. TPN generally contains KCl, multivitamins, and lipids, which do not interact with warfarin.

17. D: Patients, prescribers, and pharmacies must be registered with the Clozaril National Registry (CNR) prior to the prescription and filling of clozapine, and it is only available through a distribution system. Clozapine can cause serious agranulocytosis, rendering patients at risk for infection and death. Thus, patients require frequent monitoring of their blood counts. Clozapine is indicated for schizophrenia.

18. A: St. John's wort is often used for depression symptoms and for possible immune system benefits. Echinacea is also used for immune system support. Saw palmetto is used for benign prostatic hyperplasia, and valerian is used for its possible sedative effects. None of these agents are approved by the FDA.

19. B: Metoprolol is used for high blood pressure and tachycardia, so heart rate would be an appropriate monitoring parameter. Zoledronic acid may cause renal toxicity, so creatinine would be an appropriate monitoring parameter. Fluorouracil is an antineoplastic agent and can decrease production of white blood cells (WBCs), placing patients at risk for infection. WBCs are monitored during fluorouracil therapy. Filgrastim is used to boost neutrophils, a type of white blood cell. It does not affect triglycerides appreciably.

20. A: In certain instances, insulins may be mixed in the same syringe. Regular insulin may be mixed with NPH. Regular insulin should always be drawn up first if mixing with NPH in order to avoid the inadvertent contamination of regular insulin with NPH insulin.

21. C: Once removed, fentanyl patches should be folded together so that the sticky side sticks to itself and then flushed down the toilet in order to avoid potential danger to babies, children, or pets that might be able to access them from the trash. Unless otherwise specified (like fentanyl patches), unused prescription drugs should be removed from the bottle and mixed with an undesirable substance, such as cat litter or coffee grounds, sealed into a disposable container, and then placed in the trash.

22. A: Patients receiving rifampin should be counseled about the possibility of red-orange discoloration of urine and other body fluids, such as sweat and tears. Use may cause permanent discoloration of contact lenses. Rifampin has many drug interactions—it can increase the metabolism of many drugs, rendering them less effective. For example, rifampin can increase the metabolism of estrogens, making birth control pills less effective. It is very important that women of childbearing age who receive rifampin be counseled of this risk and the necessity of a second form of birth control.

23. D: The maximum daily dose of acetaminophen is 4,000 mg, which is 12 tablets of oxycodone/acetaminophen 5/325 (4,000 mg ÷ 325 mg ≈ 12 tablets). Patients should be counseled about the dangers of liver toxicity associated with acetaminophen use and the importance of taking the lowest effective dose. Patients should also avoid taking other agents concomitantly that may contain acetaminophen (e.g., over-the-counter medications). The Food and Drug Administration (FDA) recommended in 2009 that the maximum daily dose of acetaminophen be less than 4,000 mg due to the dangers associated with liver toxicity.

24. D: Pharmacies are notified of medication recalls by manufacturers and wholesalers by direct mail or fax. Pharmacies can also obtain recall information from the FDA website.

25. B: Digits 6 through 9 are the product code, while the first 5 digits are the manufacturer code, and the last 2 digits are the packaging code.

26. A: A Drug Enforcement Agency (DEA) number, required for each physician writing prescriptions for controlled substances, consists of two letters followed by 7 numbers. The first letter is a classification; for practitioners this letter is most commonly B or F, but may also be A or M. The second letter is the first letter of the physician's last name. To verify that the number is valid, add digits 1, 3, and 5 together. Then add digits 2, 4, and 6 together and multiply that sum by 2. Add those 2 quantities together. The result will be a two digit number, the final digit of which is called the checksum. The checksum will be the seventh number in the DEA code. In equation form, where F and S are the first and second digits in a two digit number, respectively, FS = (1st + 3rd + 5th) + 2(2nd + 4th + 6th); (2+4+3) + 2(1+6+3) = 29; 9 is final number of the DEA code.

27. C: The use of investigational drugs has many requirements in order to protect the patient. Physicians must have the approval of the institutional investigational review board (IRB) prior to drug use. Physicians must communicate risks/benefits of the investigational drug to patients and obtain signed consent. A copy of this consent must be provided to the pharmacy. The pharmacy is responsible for administrative duties, including dispensing and storage.

28. B: Two tsp is approximately 10 mL. 10 mL × 3 times daily × 7 days = 210 mL.

29. B: Because only 500 mL is required, 10 mEq of K-Phos is needed for preparation. 10 mEq ÷ 4.4 mEq/mL = 2.3 mL.

30. C: Repackaged medication labels are not required to have patient names. Generic drug name, drug strength and dose, manufacturer and lot number, and expiration date are required. Patient names are required on prescription labels.

31. D: Prescription labels must have many components, including date filled, prescription number, pharmacy address and phone number, name of physician, directions for use, and manufacturer name. Physician telephone number, date prescription written, and name of drug distributor are not required on a prescription label.

32. B: As the patient may receive 12 months of Toprol XL, and 3 months will be dispensed with the first fill, 9 months will remain on the prescription. The patient will have three refills (a 90-day supply each) remaining on the prescription.

33. A: All the choices are examples of scheduled drugs. Roxicet (C-II) is the combination of acetaminophen and oxycodone. The suffix "-et" suggests the presence of acetaminophen. Vicoprofen (C-III) is the combination of hydrocodone and ibuprofen. The suffix "-profen" suggests the presence of ibuprofen. Fiorinal (C-III) contains butalbital, aspirin, and caffeine. The suffix "-al" suggests that the product contains aspirin. Darvon (C-IV) is propoxyphene. Darvocet is the combination of propoxyphene and acetaminophen.

34. A: DEA Form 222 is used to order C-IIs. DEA Form 222 is also required for transfer of C-IIs between institutions, as one acts as the "supplier" and the other acts as the "requisitioner." DEA Form 224 is used to register a pharmacy to be able to stock controlled substances. DEA Form 41 is used to document the destruction of controlled substances. DEA Form 106 is used to document theft of controlled substances.

35. D: *N*-acetylcysteine (Mucomyst) is an antidote used for acetaminophen overdose. Vitamin K (Mephyton) is used to reverse the anticlotting effect of warfarin. Dexrazoxane (Zinecard) is used to help protect the heart from toxicity associated with anthracycline chemotherapy. It is also used for certain types of extravasations. Flumazenil (Romazicon) is used to reverse the effects of benzodiazepines.

36. B: Solid dosage forms, such as capsules, have no smell or taste, are more convenient, and easier to transport. Liquid dosage forms, however, have a faster onset of action.

37. A: Pharmacies are required to have certain equipment, including a class A balance, pharmacy weights, graduated cylinders, and mortars and pestles. Class B balances are recommended but not required.

38. C: Pharmacy technicians who work in different settings certainly have similar responsibilities, such as assisting pharmacists, prepackaging bulk medications, and maintaining inventory. Other mutual responsibilities may include training new employees and screening telephone calls. Nursing units are specific to institutions such as hospitals, and nursing inspections for outdated medications are unique to an institutional pharmacy technician.

39. D: Legally, all prescriptions, DEA forms 41 and 222, and invoices must be retrievable within 72 hours.

40. A: Dextrose 5% with sodium chloride 0.45% is commonly written as D5½NS. Dextrose 5% with sodium chloride 0.225% is commonly written as D5¼NS.

41. C: It is usually necessary to touch the syringe barrel and barrel flange when drawing up medications. One should not touch the syringe plunger, as this could contaminate the syringe. The shaft is part of the needle.

42. A: NovoLog is insulin aspart, Apidra is insulin glulisine, and Levemir is insulin detemir.

43. A: Dolophine (methadone) is a C-II. Suboxone (buprenorphine) is a C-III. Restoril (temazepam) is a C-IV. Strattera (atomoxetine) is not a controlled substance.

44. C: Fluconazole and nystatin are antifungal agents. Acyclovir is an antiviral agent. Doxycycline is an antibacterial agent.

45. C: Patanol (olopatadine) is an antihistamine eyedrop used for eye allergies.

46. C: A misbranded product has untrue or incorrect claims or labeling, including labeling that doesn't have appropriate instructions for use or warnings specific to the drug. Choices A, B, and D are examples of drug adulteration.

47. D: The prescriber must sign a prescription for a C-II. The prescription can be handwritten or typed on a computer. Patients may receive a partial fill if the remainder is available within 72 hours. Faxed C-II prescriptions are allowable from a long-term care institution. An emergency filling is allowable as long as the prescription quantity is limited to a specific time period and the physician provides the pharmacy with a hard copy within 7 days.

48. C: Although parenteral nutrition is very important, TPNs are generally not considered "stat" because patients can be maintained on IV fluids and electrolytes until TPNs are available. Cardura XL (doxazosin extended release) is a once-daily agent used for benign prostatic hyperplasia and does not have an immediate onset. A new order for Cardura XL would not be considered "stat" in a usual situation. Lotrimin (miconazole) is a topical antifungal agent, and a new order would not be considered "stat" in a usual situation. Amikacin is an antibiotic used for serious gram-negative infections and often in patients with compromised immune systems. Of the choices given, dispensing of a new order for amikacin would be considered the most pressing.

49. A: Although magnesium citrate may be tubed, it is carbonated and should be allowed to settle before opening. Many reasons exist why agents should not be tubed. Gemcitabine (Gemzar) is a chemotherapy agent and should not be tubed due to the danger of leaking and damaging the entire pneumatic tube system. Pegfilgrastim (Neulasta) should not be tubed due to the risk of protein denaturing and monetary loss if lost within the system. Abciximab (ReoPro) is also an agent that could be denatured and rendered inactive if tubed and is very expensive, making a loss very costly.

50. C: The expiration date of repackaged drugs is 6 months or 25% of the time of the manufacturer's expiration date, or whichever is less. The correct answer is 25% of 12 months, or 3 months, making the expiration 6/10.

51. C: Bupropion is Wellbutrin, olanzapine is Zyprexa, quetiapine is Seroquel, and venlafaxine is Effexor.

52. B: Abilify is aripiprazole, Cymbalta is duloxetine, Lexapro is escitalopram, and Zyprexa is olanzapine.

53. C: The type A hood exhausts a portion of the air back into the compounding room. The type B1 hood exhausts most of the air through a HEPA filter and then to the outside. The type B2 hood exhausts all air to the outside after it passes through a HEPA filter. The type B3 hood recycles air inside the hood and all exhausted air is eliminated to the outside.

54. D: The larger the gauge, the smaller the needle bore.

55. B: An FDA class I recall is the most serious, as the drug in question has a high likelihood of causing patient injury or death. An FDA class II recall is performed when a drug may cause injury that is not permanent or is treatable. An FDA class III recall is for drugs that are not likely to cause patient harm.

56. D: Tinctures, spirits, liniments, elixirs, and collodions may contain alcohol.

57. A: Silvadene is a 1% cream.

58. C: Quinine is only indicated for treatment of malaria. It has been used off label for leg cramps, but due to the risk of toxicity, it is no longer available over the counter and is not recommended for leg cramps. Quinidine, used for cardiac arrhythmias, is often mistaken for quinine.

59. D: Lioresal (baclofen) is an antispasmodic used for muscle spasms.

60. C: 2 pints = 1 quart. 4 quarts = 1 gallon. 8 pints = 1 gallon.

61. C: 1 mg = 1000 mcg. 1.33 $\times$ 1000 = 1330 mcg.

62. C: M = 1000; C = 100; L = 50; XX = 20; IV = 4. Add together for a result of 1174.

63. D: 2 tbsp = 1 fl oz; 8 fl oz = 1 cup; 16 fl oz = 2 cups; 16 fl oz $\times$ 2 tbsp/fl oz = 32 tbsp

64. D: 1 grain is approximately 65 mg. Converting mg to mcg by multiplying 65 by 1000, the answer is 65,000 mcg.

65. D: A hermetic container is airtight.

66. A: All drug choices are antineoplastic agents. Nelarabine (Arranon) is an IV agent for T-cell lymphoblastic leukemia. Vorinostat (Zolinza) is an oral agent for T-cell lymphoma. Sorafenib (Nexavar) is an oral agent for renal cell carcinoma. Erlotinib (Tarceva) is an oral agent for non-small-cell lung cancer.

67. C: The anti-inflammatory potency of prednisone is 3.0; the potency of hydrocortisone is 1.5. The potency of prednisolone, methylprednisolone, and dexamethasone are higher than prednisone at 4.0, 5.0, and 30.0, respectively.

68. D: Attention-deficit hyperactivity disorder (ADHD) is not an affective disorder but is considered a central nervous system disorder. ADHD is characterized by hyperactivity, impulsivity, and distractibility. Depression is characterized by worry, mental slowing, and sadness. Psychosis is characterized by delusions, hallucinations, and ambivalence.

69. A: The protease inhibitors, such as nelfinavir (Viracept), may cause fat redistribution. Lamivudine (Epivir) is a nucleoside reverse transcriptase inhibitor, efavirenz (Sustiva) is a nonnucleoside reverse transcriptase inhibitor, and enfuvirtide (Fuzeon) is a fusion inhibitor.

70. D: Goodman and Gilman's the Pharmacological Basis of Therapeutics is a reference for drug pharmacology and therapeutics. Remington: The Science and Practice of Pharmacy is a reference for compounding, and Handbook on Injectable Drugs ("Trissel's") is a reference for IV drug compatibility. Martindale: The Complete Drug Reference contains information about drugs worldwide.

71. C: Both Medicare and Medicaid are federally funded programs. Medicare provides health care for people age 65 and older, disabled people younger than 65 years old, and people with renal failure. Medicaid is state-administered health care for low-income individuals and families.

72. A: All patients, practitioners, and pharmacies that use isotretinoin must be registered with iPLEDGE prior to prescribing, dispensing, or administering of isotretinoin. Isotretinoin is only indicated for severe recalcitrant nodular acne. Female patients must have a monthly pregnancy test to qualify for isotretinoin prescriptions and should be counseled on the risk of teratogenicity. Patients should have a baseline triglyceride level, liver function tests, and complete blood count (CBC) prior to starting therapy and intermittently throughout therapy. Patients should be counseled on the risk of psychiatric disorders, which have occurred in patients taking isotretinoin, including severe depression and suicidality.

73. C: 0.5% = 0.005; 10 gm × 0.005 = 0.05 g or 50 mg.

74. C: Convert both to milligrams (300 mcg = 0.3 mg; 3 gm = 3,000 mg). Then divide 3,000 mg by 0.3 mg for a result of 10,000 tablets.

75. B: The original and transferred prescriptions must be kept on file for at least two years.

76. C: Both K-Lor and KCL are oral products. K-Lor must be diluted prior to delivery, and a child is likely to spit out or refuse K-Lor or KCl oral solution medications. K-Dur is a solid dosage form too large for a child to take. A KCl IV piggyback would provide the most accurate dose.

77. B: 5% of $114 is calculated by multiplying 114 by 0.05 for a result (discount) of $5.70. $5.70 subtracted from $114.00 is $108.30.

78. C: The higher the turnover rate, the better the financial health of an institution. Twelve is considered a turnover rate that is very good. Inventory turnover rate is calculated by total annual purchases divided by the value of inventory.

79. D: Only institutions with a Drug Enforcement Agency (DEA) number can return controlled substances. A DEA Form 41 must be completed and submitted to the DEA prior to the destruction of controlled substances. A copy of this form must be maintained on file for at least two years. DEA Form 222 is for the purchasing or transferring of controlled substances.

80. B: A group purchasing organization negotiates with drug manufacturers for reduced medication prices on behalf of health-care institutions and makes contracts with these companies. The health-care institution purchases medications, not the group purchasing organization.

81. D: A formulary is a list of medications that has been approved for use in a health-care institution. The pharmacy and therapeutics (P&T) committee makes the formulary, and its members include pharmacists, physicians, nurses, and those involved with the purchasing of pharmaceuticals.

82. A: Therapeutic substitution is the process by which a drug has been deemed to have similar therapeutic activity and pharmacokinetics to another drug, despite differences in composition—these drugs may be interchanged. Therapeutic equivalency is when a drug is considered the same as another drug due to similarities in therapeutic activity and pharmacokinetics. Bioavailability is the absorption, distribution, metabolism, and elimination of a drug. Therapeutic equality is not a term used in pharmacy.

83. D: Jewelry should not be worn when compounding due to the risk of contaminating the sterile field and product. Gloves will not eliminate this risk. Makeup should not be worn due to the risk of particulate dispersal from the makeup. A mask will not eliminate this risk. Hands should be washed prior to donning gloves and at routine intervals during compounding. Compounding gowns are recommended to reduce the release of particulate matter.

84. D: The DEA enforces the Controlled Substances Act. State boards of pharmacy monitor pharmacist licensure, technician requirements, and pharmacy permits. The Joint Commission ensures that institutional pharmacies prepare and dispense unit dose medications and patient-specific IV medications. The United States Pharmacopeia makes rules regarding the labeling of medications.

85. D: According to the Institute for Safe Medication Practices (ISMP), drug name suffixes can lead to confusion and medication error. Errors have occurred, such as the dispensing of the wrong drug and wrong dose. Extra precautions should be implemented when filling prescriptions with suffixes in order to ensure that the correct drug and/or dosage form is being supplied to the patient. Any confusion should be clarified with the prescriber before dispensing. Imodium A-D is an oral antidiarrheal. Procardia XL is an oral antihypertensive agent. Diprolene AF is a topical corticosteroid.

86. A: The U.S. Department of Transportation makes regulations regarding the shipping of hazardous materials, which pertains to radiopharmaceuticals. Radioactive Yellow III material contains the highest concentration of radiation compared to Radioactive Yellow I and II. A special metal shipping container is required for transportation, and a special placard must be placed on any vehicle transporting such an agent.

87. D: HEPA stands for high-efficiency particulate air. It prevents particles greater than three microns from entering the sterile environment. Cleaning agents, such as 70% alcohol, should not be sprayed on the filter due to the risk of causing holes. The hood should be certified anytime the HEPA filter becomes wet.

88. C: Tonicity is the measure of osmotic pressure. A hypertonic solution pulls fluid out of cells. Three percent sodium chloride is considered hypertonic. A hypotonic solution draws water into cells, which can cause cells to burst. Water is hypotonic, and plain water (i.e., water without additives) MUST NEVER be hung intravenously or peripherally on patients. Normal saline (0.9%) is isotonic, which does not pull water into or out of cells.

89. C: Rubber spatulas are used for corrosive agents. Digital balances are sensitive to 0.01 mg. Glass mortars and pestles are used for mixing liquid and semisolid agents. TD ("to deliver") graduated cylinders deliver the exact amount, while TC ("to contain") graduated cylinders do not deliver the exact amount due to the residue left in the cylinder.

90. C: The Omnibus Reconciliation Budget Reconciliation Act of 1990 (OBRA 90) requires that pharmacists perform drug utilization reviews (DUEs) and maintain patient profiles. A medication administration record (MAR) is used by the nursing staff to record drug delivery to patients. The Americans with Disabilities Act (ADA) requires that businesses do not discriminate against the disabled.

How to Overcome Test Anxiety

Just the thought of taking a test is enough to make most people a little nervous. A test is an important event that can have a long-term impact on your future, so it's important to take it seriously and it's natural to feel anxious about performing well. But just because anxiety is normal, that doesn't mean that it's helpful in test taking, or that you should simply accept it as part of your life. Anxiety can have a variety of effects. These effects can be mild, like making you feel slightly nervous, or severe, like blocking your ability to focus or remember even a simple detail.

If you experience test anxiety—whether severe or mild—it's important to know how to beat it. To discover this, first you need to understand what causes test anxiety.

Causes of Test Anxiety

While we often think of anxiety as an uncontrollable emotional state, it can actually be caused by simple, practical things. One of the most common causes of test anxiety is that a person does not feel adequately prepared for their test. This feeling can be the result of many different issues such as poor study habits or lack of organization, but the most common culprit is time management. Starting to study too late, failing to organize your study time to cover all of the material, or being distracted while you study will mean that you're not well prepared for the test. This may lead to cramming the night before, which will cause you to be physically and mentally exhausted for the test. Poor time management also contributes to feelings of stress, fear, and hopelessness as you realize you are not well prepared but don't know what to do about it.

Other times, test anxiety is not related to your preparation for the test but comes from unresolved fear. This may be a past failure on a test, or poor performance on tests in general. It may come from comparing yourself to others who seem to be performing better or from the stress of living up to expectations. Anxiety may be driven by fears of the future—how failure on this test would affect your educational and career goals. These fears are often completely irrational, but they can still negatively impact your test performance.

Review Video: 3 Reasons You Have Test Anxiety
Visit mometrix.com/academy and enter code: 428468

Elements of Test Anxiety

As mentioned earlier, test anxiety is considered to be an emotional state, but it has physical and mental components as well. Sometimes you may not even realize that you are suffering from test anxiety until you notice the physical symptoms. These can include trembling hands, rapid heartbeat, sweating, nausea, and tense muscles. Extreme anxiety may lead to fainting or vomiting. Obviously, any of these symptoms can have a negative impact on testing. It is important to recognize them as soon as they begin to occur so that you can address the problem before it damages your performance.

Review Video: 3 Ways to Tell You Have Test Anxiety
Visit mometrix.com/academy and enter code: 927847

The mental components of test anxiety include trouble focusing and inability to remember learned information. During a test, your mind is on high alert, which can help you recall information and stay focused for an extended period of time. However, anxiety interferes with your mind's natural processes, causing you to blank out, even on the questions you know well. The strain of testing during anxiety makes it difficult to stay focused, especially on a test that may take several hours. Extreme anxiety can take a huge mental toll, making it difficult not only to recall test information but even to understand the test questions or pull your thoughts together.

Review Video: How Test Anxiety Affects Memory
Visit mometrix.com/academy and enter code: 609003

Effects of Test Anxiety

Test anxiety is like a disease—if left untreated, it will get progressively worse. Anxiety leads to poor performance, and this reinforces the feelings of fear and failure, which in turn lead to poor performances on subsequent tests. It can grow from a mild nervousness to a crippling condition. If allowed to progress, test anxiety can have a big impact on your schooling, and consequently on your future.

Test anxiety can spread to other parts of your life. Anxiety on tests can become anxiety in any stressful situation, and blanking on a test can turn into panicking in a job situation. But fortunately, you don't have to let anxiety rule your testing and determine your grades. There are a number of relatively simple steps you can take to move past anxiety and function normally on a test and in the rest of life.

Review Video: How Test Anxiety Impacts Your Grades
Visit mometrix.com/academy and enter code: 939819

Physical Steps for Beating Test Anxiety

While test anxiety is a serious problem, the good news is that it can be overcome. It doesn't have to control your ability to think and remember information. While it may take time, you can begin taking steps today to beat anxiety.

Just as your first hint that you may be struggling with anxiety comes from the physical symptoms, the first step to treating it is also physical. Rest is crucial for having a clear, strong mind. If you are tired, it is much easier to give in to anxiety. But if you establish good sleep habits, your body and mind will be ready to perform optimally, without the strain of exhaustion. Additionally, sleeping well helps you to retain information better, so you're more likely to recall the answers when you see the test questions.

Getting good sleep means more than going to bed on time. It's important to allow your brain time to relax. Take study breaks from time to time so it doesn't get overworked, and don't study right before bed. Take time to rest your mind before trying to rest your body, or you may find it difficult to fall asleep.

Review Video: The Importance of Sleep for Your Brain
Visit mometrix.com/academy and enter code: 319338

Along with sleep, other aspects of physical health are important in preparing for a test. Good nutrition is vital for good brain function. Sugary foods and drinks may give a burst of energy but this burst is followed by a crash, both physically and emotionally. Instead, fuel your body with protein and vitamin-rich foods.

Also, drink plenty of water. Dehydration can lead to headaches and exhaustion, especially if your brain is already under stress from the rigors of the test. Particularly if your test is a long one, drink water during the breaks. And if possible, take an energy-boosting snack to eat between sections.

Review Video: How Diet Can Affect your Mood
Visit mometrix.com/academy and enter code: 624317

Along with sleep and diet, a third important part of physical health is exercise. Maintaining a steady workout schedule is helpful, but even taking 5-minute study breaks to walk can help get your blood pumping faster and clear your head. Exercise also releases endorphins, which contribute to a positive feeling and can help combat test anxiety.

When you nurture your physical health, you are also contributing to your mental health. If your body is healthy, your mind is much more likely to be healthy as well. So take time to rest, nourish your body with healthy food and water, and get moving as much as possible. Taking these physical steps will make you stronger and more able to take the mental steps necessary to overcome test anxiety.

Review Video: How to Stay Healthy and Prevent Test Anxiety
Visit mometrix.com/academy and enter code: 877894

Mental Steps for Beating Test Anxiety

Working on the mental side of test anxiety can be more challenging, but as with the physical side, there are clear steps you can take to overcome it. As mentioned earlier, test anxiety often stems from lack of preparation, so the obvious solution is to prepare for the test. Effective studying may be the most important weapon you have for beating test anxiety, but you can and should employ several other mental tools to combat fear.

First, boost your confidence by reminding yourself of past success—tests or projects that you aced. If you're putting as much effort into preparing for this test as you did for those, there's no reason you should expect to fail here. Work hard to prepare; then trust your preparation.

Second, surround yourself with encouraging people. It can be helpful to find a study group, but be sure that the people you're around will encourage a positive attitude. If you spend time with others who are anxious or cynical, this will only contribute to your own anxiety. Look for others who are motivated to study hard from a desire to succeed, not from a fear of failure.

Third, reward yourself. A test is physically and mentally tiring, even without anxiety, and it can be helpful to have something to look forward to. Plan an activity following the test, regardless of the outcome, such as going to a movie or getting ice cream.

When you are taking the test, if you find yourself beginning to feel anxious, remind yourself that you know the material. Visualize successfully completing the test. Then take a few deep, relaxing breaths and return to it. Work through the questions carefully but with confidence, knowing that you are capable of succeeding.

Developing a healthy mental approach to test taking will also aid in other areas of life. Test anxiety affects more than just the actual test—it can be damaging to your mental health and even contribute to depression. It's important to beat test anxiety before it becomes a problem for more than testing.

Review Video: Test Anxiety and Depression
Visit mometrix.com/academy and enter code: 904704

Study Strategy

Being prepared for the test is necessary to combat anxiety, but what does being prepared look like? You may study for hours on end and still not feel prepared. What you need is a strategy for test prep. The next few pages outline our recommended steps to help you plan out and conquer the challenge of preparation.

Step 1: Scope Out the Test

Learn everything you can about the format (multiple choice, essay, etc.) and what will be on the test. Gather any study materials, course outlines, or sample exams that may be available. Not only will this help you to prepare, but knowing what to expect can help to alleviate test anxiety.

Step 2: Map Out the Material

Look through the textbook or study guide and make note of how many chapters or sections it has. Then divide these over the time you have. For example, if a book has 15 chapters and you have five days to study, you need to cover three chapters each day. Even better, if you have the time, leave an extra day at the end for overall review after you have gone through the material in depth.

If time is limited, you may need to prioritize the material. Look through it and make note of which sections you think you already have a good grasp on, and which need review. While you are studying, skim quickly through the familiar sections and take more time on the challenging parts. Write out your plan so you don't get lost as you go. Having a written plan also helps you feel more in control of the study, so anxiety is less likely to arise from feeling overwhelmed at the amount to cover. A sample plan may look like this:

- Day 1: Skim chapters 1–4, study chapter 5 (especially pages 31–33)
- Day 2: Study chapters 6–7, skim chapters 8–9
- Day 3: Skim chapter 10, study chapters 11–12 (especially pages 87–90)
- Day 4: Study chapters 13–15
- Day 5: Overall review (focus most on chapters 5, 6, and 12), take practice test

Step 3: Gather Your Tools

Decide what study method works best for you. Do you prefer to highlight in the book as you study and then go back over the highlighted portions? Or do you type out notes of the important information? Or is it helpful to make flashcards that you can carry with you? Assemble the pens, index cards, highlighters, post-it notes, and any other materials you may need so you won't be distracted by getting up to find things while you study.

If you're having a hard time retaining the information or organizing your notes, experiment with different methods. For example, try color-coding by subject with colored pens, highlighters, or post-it notes. If you learn better by hearing, try recording yourself reading your notes so you can listen while in the car, working out, or simply sitting at your desk. Ask a friend to quiz you from your flashcards, or try teaching someone the material to solidify it in your mind.

Step 4: Create Your Environment

It's important to avoid distractions while you study. This includes both the obvious distractions like visitors and the subtle distractions like an uncomfortable chair (or a too-comfortable couch that makes you want to fall asleep). Set up the best study environment possible: good lighting and a comfortable work area. If background music helps you focus, you may want to turn it on, but otherwise keep the room quiet. If you are using a computer to take notes, be sure you don't have any other windows open, especially applications like social media, games, or anything else that could distract you. Silence your phone and turn off notifications. Be sure to keep water close by so you stay hydrated while you study (but avoid unhealthy drinks and snacks).

Also, take into account the best time of day to study. Are you freshest first thing in the morning? Try to set aside some time then to work through the material. Is your mind clearer in the afternoon or evening? Schedule your study session then. Another method is to study at the same time of day that you will take the test, so that your brain gets used to working on the material at that time and will be ready to focus at test time.

STEP 5: STUDY!

Once you have done all the study preparation, it's time to settle into the actual studying. Sit down, take a few moments to settle your mind so you can focus, and begin to follow your study plan. Don't give in to distractions or let yourself procrastinate. This is your time to prepare so you'll be ready to fearlessly approach the test. Make the most of the time and stay focused.

Of course, you don't want to burn out. If you study too long you may find that you're not retaining the information very well. Take regular study breaks. For example, taking five minutes out of every hour to walk briskly, breathing deeply and swinging your arms, can help your mind stay fresh.

As you get to the end of each chapter or section, it's a good idea to do a quick review. Remind yourself of what you learned and work on any difficult parts. When you feel that you've mastered the material, move on to the next part. At the end of your study session, briefly skim through your notes again.

But while review is helpful, cramming last minute is NOT. If at all possible, work ahead so that you won't need to fit all your study into the last day. Cramming overloads your brain with more information than it can process and retain, and your tired mind may struggle to recall even previously learned information when it is overwhelmed with last-minute study. Also, the urgent nature of cramming and the stress placed on your brain contribute to anxiety. You'll be more likely to go to the test feeling unprepared and having trouble thinking clearly.

So don't cram, and don't stay up late before the test, even just to review your notes at a leisurely pace. Your brain needs rest more than it needs to go over the information again. In fact, plan to finish your studies by noon or early afternoon the day before the test. Give your brain the rest of the day to relax or focus on other things, and get a good night's sleep. Then you will be fresh for the test and better able to recall what you've studied.

STEP 6: TAKE A PRACTICE TEST

Many courses offer sample tests, either online or in the study materials. This is an excellent resource to check whether you have mastered the material, as well as to prepare for the test format and environment.

Check the test format ahead of time: the number of questions, the type (multiple choice, free response, etc.), and the time limit. Then create a plan for working through them. For example, if you have 30 minutes to take a 60-question test, your limit is 30 seconds per question. Spend less time on the questions you know well so that you can take more time on the difficult ones.

If you have time to take several practice tests, take the first one open book, with no time limit. Work through the questions at your own pace and make sure you fully understand them. Gradually work up to taking a test under test conditions: sit at a desk with all study materials put away and set a timer. Pace yourself to make sure you finish the test with time to spare and go back to check your answers if you have time.

After each test, check your answers. On the questions you missed, be sure you understand why you missed them. Did you misread the question (tests can use tricky wording)? Did you forget the information? Or was it something you hadn't learned? Go back and study any shaky areas that the practice tests reveal.

Taking these tests not only helps with your grade, but also aids in combating test anxiety. If you're already used to the test conditions, you're less likely to worry about it, and working through tests until you're scoring well gives you a confidence boost. Go through the practice tests until you feel comfortable, and then you can go into the test knowing that you're ready for it.

Test Tips

On test day, you should be confident, knowing that you've prepared well and are ready to answer the questions. But aside from preparation, there are several test day strategies you can employ to maximize your performance.

First, as stated before, get a good night's sleep the night before the test (and for several nights before that, if possible). Go into the test with a fresh, alert mind rather than staying up late to study.

Try not to change too much about your normal routine on the day of the test. It's important to eat a nutritious breakfast, but if you normally don't eat breakfast at all, consider eating just a protein bar. If you're a coffee drinker, go ahead and have your normal coffee. Just make sure you time it so that the caffeine doesn't wear off right in the middle of your test. Avoid sugary beverages, and drink enough water to stay hydrated but not so much that you need a restroom break 10 minutes into the test. If your test isn't first thing in the morning, consider going for a walk or doing a light workout before the test to get your blood flowing.

Allow yourself enough time to get ready, and leave for the test with plenty of time to spare so you won't have the anxiety of scrambling to arrive in time. Another reason to be early is to select a good seat. It's helpful to sit away from doors and windows, which can be distracting. Find a good seat, get out your supplies, and settle your mind before the test begins.

When the test begins, start by going over the instructions carefully, even if you already know what to expect. Make sure you avoid any careless mistakes by following the directions.

Then begin working through the questions, pacing yourself as you've practiced. If you're not sure on an answer, don't spend too much time on it, and don't let it shake your confidence. Either skip it and come back later, or eliminate as many wrong answers as possible and guess among the remaining ones. Don't dwell on these questions as you continue—put them out of your mind and focus on what lies ahead.

Be sure to read all of the answer choices, even if you're sure the first one is the right answer. Sometimes you'll find a better one if you keep reading. But don't second-guess yourself if you do immediately know the answer. Your gut instinct is usually right. Don't let test anxiety rob you of the information you know.

If you have time at the end of the test (and if the test format allows), go back and review your answers. Be cautious about changing any, since your first instinct tends to be correct, but make sure you didn't misread any of the questions or accidentally mark the wrong answer choice. Look over any you skipped and make an educated guess.

At the end, leave the test feeling confident. You've done your best, so don't waste time worrying about your performance or wishing you could change anything. Instead, celebrate the successful completion of this test. And finally, use this test to learn how to deal with anxiety even better next time.

Review Video: 5 Tips to Beat Test Anxiety
Visit mometrix.com/academy and enter code: 570656

Important Qualification

Not all anxiety is created equal. If your test anxiety is causing major issues in your life beyond the classroom or testing center, or if you are experiencing troubling physical symptoms related to your anxiety, it may be a sign of a serious physiological or psychological condition. If this sounds like your situation, we strongly encourage you to seek professional help.

How to Overcome Your Fear of Math

The word *math* is enough to strike fear into most hearts. How many of us have memories of sitting through confusing lectures, wrestling over mind-numbing homework, or taking tests that still seem incomprehensible even after hours of study? Years after graduation, many still shudder at these memories.

The fact is, math is not just a classroom subject. It has real-world implications that you face every day, whether you realize it or not. This may be balancing your monthly budget, deciding how many supplies to buy for a project, or simply splitting a meal check with friends. The idea of daily confrontations with math can be so paralyzing that some develop a condition known as *math anxiety*.

But you do NOT need to be paralyzed by this anxiety! In fact, while you may have thought all your life that you're not good at math, or that your brain isn't wired to understand it, the truth is that you may have been conditioned to think this way. From your earliest school days, the way you were taught affected the way you viewed different subjects. And the way math has been taught has changed.

Several decades ago, there was a shift in American math classrooms. The focus changed from traditional problem-solving to a conceptual view of topics, de-emphasizing the importance of learning the basics and building on them. The solid foundation necessary for math progression and confidence was undermined. Math became more of a vague concept than a concrete idea. Today, it is common to think of math, not as a straightforward system, but as a mysterious, complicated method that can't be fully understood unless you're a genius.

This is why you may still have nightmares about being called on to answer a difficult problem in front of the class. Math anxiety is a very real, though unnecessary, fear.

Math anxiety may begin with a single class period. Let's say you missed a day in 6th grade math and never quite understood the concept that was taught while you were gone. Since math is cumulative, with each new concept building on past ones, this could very well affect the rest of your math career. Without that one day's knowledge, it will be difficult to understand any other concepts that link to it. Rather than realizing that you're just missing one key piece, you may begin to believe that you're simply not capable of understanding math.

This belief can change the way you approach other classes, career options, and everyday life experiences, if you become anxious at the thought that math might be required. A student who loves science may choose a different path of study upon realizing that multiple math classes will be required for a degree. An aspiring medical student may hesitate at the thought of going through the necessary math classes. For some this anxiety escalates into a more extreme state known as *math phobia*.

Math anxiety is challenging to address because it is rooted deeply and may come from a variety of causes: an embarrassing moment in class, a teacher who did not explain concepts well and contributed to a shaky foundation, or a failed test that contributed to the belief of math failure.

These causes add up over time, encouraged by society's popular view that math is hard and unpleasant. Eventually a person comes to firmly believe that he or she is simply bad at math. This belief makes it difficult to grasp new concepts or even remember old ones. Homework and test grades begin to slip, which only confirms the belief. The poor performance is not due to lack of ability but is caused by math anxiety.

Math anxiety is an emotional issue, not a lack of intelligence. But when it becomes deeply rooted, it can become more than just an emotional problem. Physical symptoms appear. Blood pressure may rise and heartbeat may quicken at the sight of a math problem – or even the thought of math! This fear leads to a mental block. When someone with math anxiety is asked to perform a calculation, even a basic problem can seem overwhelming and impossible. The emotional and physical response to the thought of math prevents the brain from working through it logically.

The more this happens, the more a person's confidence drops, and the more math anxiety is generated. This vicious cycle must be broken!

The first step in breaking the cycle is to go back to very beginning and make sure you really understand the basics of how math works and why it works. It is not enough to memorize rules for multiplication and division. If you don't know WHY these rules work, your foundation will be shaky and you will be at risk of developing a phobia. Understanding mathematical concepts not only promotes confidence and security, but allows you to build on this understanding for new concepts. Additionally, you can solve unfamiliar problems using familiar concepts and processes.

Why is it that students in other countries regularly outperform American students in math? The answer likely boils down to a couple of things: the foundation of mathematical conceptual understanding and societal perception. While students in the US are not expected to *like* or *get* math, in many other nations, students are expected not only to understand math but also to excel at it.

Changing the American view of math that leads to math anxiety is a monumental task. It requires changing the training of teachers nationwide, from kindergarten through high school, so that they learn to teach the *why* behind math and to combat the wrong math views that students may develop. It also involves changing the stigma associated with math, so that it is no longer viewed as unpleasant and incomprehensible. While these are necessary changes, they are challenging and will take time. But in the meantime, math anxiety is not irreversible—it can be faced and defeated, one person at a time.

False Beliefs

One reason math anxiety has taken such hold is that several false beliefs have been created and shared until they became widely accepted. Some of these unhelpful beliefs include the following:

There is only one way to solve a math problem. In the same way that you can choose from different driving routes and still arrive at the same house, you can solve a math problem using different methods and still find the correct answer. A person who understands the reasoning behind math calculations may be able to look at an unfamiliar concept and find the right answer, just by applying logic to the knowledge they already have. This approach may be different than what is taught in the classroom, but it is still valid. Unfortunately, even many teachers view math as a subject where the best course of action is to memorize the rule or process for each problem rather than as a place for students to exercise logic and creativity in finding a solution.

Many people don't have a mind for math. A person who has struggled due to poor teaching or math anxiety may falsely believe that he or she doesn't have the mental capacity to grasp mathematical concepts. Most of the time, this is false. Many people find that when they are relieved of their math anxiety, they have more than enough brainpower to understand math.

Men are naturally better at math than women. Even though research has shown this to be false, many young women still avoid math careers and classes because of their belief that their math abilities are inferior. Many girls have come to believe that math is a male skill and have given up trying to understand or enjoy it.

Counting aids are bad. Something like counting on your fingers or drawing out a problem to visualize it may be frowned on as childish or a crutch, but these devices can help you get a tangible understanding of a problem or a concept.

Sadly, many students buy into these ideologies at an early age. A young girl who enjoys math class may be conditioned to think that she doesn't actually have the brain for it because math is for boys, and may turn her energies to other pursuits, permanently closing the door on a wide range of opportunities. A child who finds the right answer but doesn't follow the teacher's method may believe that he is doing it wrong and isn't good at math. A student who never had a problem with math before may have a poor teacher and become confused, yet believe that the problem is because she doesn't have a mathematical mind.

Students who have bought into these erroneous beliefs quickly begin to add their own anxieties, adapting them to their own personal situations:

I'll never use this in real life. A huge number of people wrongly believe that math is irrelevant outside the classroom. By adopting this mindset, they are handicapping themselves for a life in a mathematical world, as well as limiting their career choices. When they are inevitably faced with real-world math, they are conditioning themselves to respond with anxiety.

I'm not quick enough. While timed tests and quizzes, or even simply comparing yourself with other students in the class, can lead to this belief, speed is not an indicator of skill level. A person can work very slowly yet understand at a deep level.

If I can understand it, it's too easy. People with a low view of their own abilities tend to think that if they are able to grasp a concept, it must be simple. They cannot accept the idea that they are capable of understanding math. This belief will make it harder to learn, no matter how intelligent they are.

I just can't learn this. An overwhelming number of people think this, from young children to adults, and much of the time it is simply not true. But this mindset can turn into a self-fulfilling prophecy that keeps you from exercising and growing your math ability.

The good news is, each of these myths can be debunked. For most people, they are based on emotion and psychology, NOT on actual ability! It will take time, effort, and the desire to change, but change is possible. Even if you have spent years thinking that you don't have the capability to understand math, it is not too late to uncover your true ability and find relief from the anxiety that surrounds math.

Math Strategies

It is important to have a plan of attack to combat math anxiety. There are many useful strategies for pinpointing the fears or myths and eradicating them:

Go back to the basics. For most people, math anxiety stems from a poor foundation. You may think that you have a complete understanding of addition and subtraction, or even decimals and percentages, but make absolutely sure. Learning math is different from learning other subjects. For example, when you learn history, you study various time periods and places and events. It may be important to memorize dates or find out about the lives of famous people. When you move from US history to world history, there will be some overlap, but a large amount of the information will be new. Mathematical concepts, on the other hand, are very closely linked and highly dependent on each other. It's like climbing a ladder – if a rung is missing from your understanding, it may be difficult or impossible for you to climb any higher, no matter how hard you try. So go back and make sure your math foundation is strong. This may mean taking a remedial math course, going to a tutor to work through the shaky concepts, or just going through your old homework to make sure you really understand it.

Speak the language. Math has a large vocabulary of terms and phrases unique to working problems. Sometimes these are completely new terms, and sometimes they are common words, but are used differently in a math setting. If you can't speak the language, it will be very difficult to get a thorough understanding of the concepts. It's common for students to think that they don't understand math when they simply don't understand the vocabulary. The good news is that this is fairly easy to fix. Brushing up on any terms you aren't quite sure of can help bring the rest of the concepts into focus.

Check your anxiety level. When you think about math, do you feel nervous or uncomfortable? Do you struggle with feelings of inadequacy, even on concepts that you know you've already learned? It's important to understand your specific math anxieties, and what triggers them. When you catch yourself falling back on a false belief, mentally replace it with the truth. Don't let yourself believe that you can't learn, or that struggling with a concept means you'll never understand it. Instead, remind yourself of how much you've already learned and dwell on that past success. Visualize grasping the new concept, linking it to your old knowledge, and moving on to the next challenge. Also, learn how to manage anxiety when it arises. There are many techniques for coping with the irrational fears that rise to the surface when you enter the math classroom. This may include controlled breathing, replacing negative thoughts with positive ones, or visualizing success. Anxiety interferes with your ability to concentrate and absorb information, which in turn contributes to greater anxiety. If you can learn how to regain control of your thinking, you will be better able to pay attention, make progress, and succeed!

Don't go it alone. Like any deeply ingrained belief, math anxiety is not easy to eradicate. And there is no need for you to wrestle through it on your own. It will take time, and many people find that speaking with a counselor or psychiatrist helps. They can help you develop strategies for responding to anxiety and overcoming old ideas. Additionally, it can be very helpful to take a short course or seek out a math tutor to help you find and fix the missing rungs on your ladder and make sure that you're ready to progress to the next level. You can also find a number of math aids online: courses that will teach you mental devices for figuring out problems, how to get the most out of your math classes, etc.

Check your math attitude. No matter how much you want to learn and overcome your anxiety, you'll have trouble if you still have a negative attitude toward math. If you think it's too hard, or just have general feelings of dread about math, it will be hard to learn and to break through the anxiety. Work on cultivating a positive math attitude. Remind yourself that math is not just a hurdle to be cleared, but a valuable asset. When you view math with a positive attitude, you'll be much more likely to understand and even enjoy it. This is something you must do for yourself. You may find it helpful to visit with a counselor. Your tutor, friends, and family may cheer you on in your endeavors. But your greatest asset is yourself. You are inside your own mind – tell yourself what you need to hear. Relive past victories. Remind yourself that you are capable of understanding math. Root out any false beliefs that linger and replace them with positive truths. Even if it doesn't feel true at first, it will begin to affect your thinking and pave the way for a positive, anxiety-free mindset.

Aside from these general strategies, there are a number of specific practical things you can do to begin your journey toward overcoming math anxiety. Something as simple as learning a new note-taking strategy can change the way you approach math and give you more confidence and understanding. New study techniques can also make a huge difference.

Math anxiety leads to bad habits. If it causes you to be afraid of answering a question in class, you may gravitate toward the back row. You may be embarrassed to ask for help. And you may procrastinate on assignments, which leads to rushing through them at the last moment when it's too late to get a better understanding. It's important to identify your negative behaviors and replace them with positive ones:

Prepare ahead of time. Read the lesson before you go to class. Being exposed to the topics that will be covered in class ahead of time, even if you don't understand them perfectly, is extremely helpful in increasing what you retain from the lecture. Do your homework and, if you're still shaky, go over some extra problems. The key to a solid understanding of math is practice.

Sit front and center. When you can easily see and hear, you'll understand more, and you'll avoid the distractions of other students if no one is in front of you. Plus, you're more likely to be sitting with students who are positive and engaged, rather than others with math anxiety. Let their positive math attitude rub off on you.

Ask questions in class and out. If you don't understand something, just ask. If you need a more in-depth explanation, the teacher may need to work with you outside of class, but often it's a simple concept you don't quite understand, and a single question may clear it up. If you wait, you may not be able to follow the rest of the day's lesson. For extra help, most professors have office hours outside of class when you can go over concepts one-on-one to clear up any uncertainties. Additionally, there may be a *math lab* or study session you can attend for homework help. Take advantage of this.

Review. Even if you feel that you've fully mastered a concept, review it periodically to reinforce it. Going over an old lesson has several benefits: solidifying your understanding, giving you a confidence boost, and even giving some new insights into material that you're currently learning! Don't let yourself get rusty. That can lead to problems with learning later concepts.

Teaching Tips

While the math student's mindset is the most crucial to overcoming math anxiety, it is also important for others to adjust their math attitudes. Teachers and parents have an enormous influence on how students relate to math. They can either contribute to math confidence or math anxiety.

As a parent or teacher, it is very important to convey a positive math attitude. Retelling horror stories of your own bad experience with math will contribute to a new generation of math anxiety. Even if you don't share your experiences, others will be able to sense your fears and may begin to believe them.

Even a careless comment can have a big impact, so watch for phrases like *He's not good at math* or *I never liked math*. You are a crucial role model, and your children or students will unconsciously adopt your mindset. Give them a positive example to follow. Rather than teaching them to fear the math world before they even know it, teach them about all its potential and excitement.

Work to present math as an integral, beautiful, and understandable part of life. Encourage creativity in solving problems. Watch for false beliefs and dispel them. Cross the lines between subjects: integrate history, English, and music with math. Show students how math is used every day, and how the entire world is based on mathematical principles, from the pull of gravity to the shape of seashells. Instead of letting students see math as a necessary evil, direct them to view it as an imaginative, beautiful art form – an art form that they are capable of mastering and using.

Don't give too narrow a view of math. It is more than just numbers. Yes, working problems and learning formulas is a large part of classroom math. But don't let the teaching stop there. Teach students about the everyday implications of math. Show them how nature works according to the laws of mathematics, and take them outside to make discoveries of their own. Expose them to math-related careers by inviting visiting speakers, asking students to do research and presentations, and learning students' interests and aptitudes on a personal level.

Demonstrate the importance of math. Many people see math as nothing more than a required stepping stone to their degree, a nuisance with no real usefulness. Teach students that algebra is used every day in managing their bank accounts, in following recipes, and in scheduling the day's events. Show them how learning to do geometric proofs helps them to develop logical thinking, an invaluable life skill. Let them see that math surrounds them and is integrally linked to their daily lives: that weather predictions are based on math, that math was used to design cars and other machines, etc. Most of all, give them the tools to use math to enrich their lives.

Make math as tangible as possible. Use visual aids and objects that can be touched. It is much easier to grasp a concept when you can hold it in your hands and manipulate it, rather than just listening to the lecture. Encourage math outside of the classroom. The real world is full of measuring, counting, and calculating, so let students participate in this. Keep your eyes open for numbers and patterns to discuss. Talk about how scores are calculated in sports games and how far apart plants are placed in a garden row for maximum growth. Build the mindset that math is a normal and interesting part of daily life.

Finally, find math resources that help to build a positive math attitude. There are a number of books that show math as fascinating and exciting while teaching important concepts, for example: *The Math Curse; A Wrinkle in Time; The Phantom Tollbooth;* and *Fractals, Googols and Other Mathematical Tales*. You can also find a number of online resources: math puzzles and games, videos that show math in nature, and communities of math enthusiasts. On a local level, students can compete in a variety of math competitions with other schools or join a math club.

The student who experiences math as exciting and interesting is unlikely to suffer from math anxiety. Going through life without this handicap is an immense advantage and opens many doors that others have closed through their fear.

Self-Check

Whether you suffer from math anxiety or not, chances are that you have been exposed to some of the false beliefs mentioned above. Now is the time to check yourself for any errors you may have accepted. Do you think you're not wired for math? Or that you don't need to understand it since you're not planning on a math career? Do you think math is just too difficult for the average person?

Find the errors you've taken to heart and replace them with positive thinking. Are you capable of learning math? Yes! Can you control your anxiety? Yes! These errors will resurface from time to time, so be watchful. Don't let others with math anxiety influence you or sway your confidence. If you're having trouble with a concept, find help. Don't let it discourage you!

Create a plan of attack for defeating math anxiety and sharpening your skills. Do some research and decide if it would help you to take a class, get a tutor, or find some online resources to fine-tune your knowledge. Make the effort to get good nutrition, hydration, and sleep so that you are operating at full capacity. Remind yourself daily that you are skilled and that anxiety does not control you. Your mind is capable of so much more than you know. Give it the tools it needs to grow and thrive.

Thank You

We at Mometrix would like to extend our heartfelt thanks to you, our friend and patron, for allowing us to play a part in your journey. It is a privilege to serve people from all walks of life who are unified in their commitment to building the best future they can for themselves.

The preparation you devote to these important testing milestones may be the most valuable educational opportunity you have for making a real difference in your life. We encourage you to put your heart into it—that feeling of succeeding, overcoming, and yes, conquering will be well worth the hours you've invested.

We want to hear your story, your struggles and your successes, and if you see any opportunities for us to improve our materials so we can help others even more effectively in the future, please share that with us as well. **The team at Mometrix would be absolutely thrilled to hear from you!** So please, send us an email (support@mometrix.com) and let's stay in touch.

If you'd like some additional help, check out these other resources we offer for your exam: http://MometrixFlashcards.com/PTCB

Additional Bonus Material

Due to our efforts to try to keep this book to a manageable length, we've created a link that will give you access to all of your additional bonus material.

Please visit https://www.mometrix.com/bonus948/ptcb to access the information.

Made in the USA
San Bernardino, CA
01 September 2019